ADVANCED
AROMATHERAPY

ADVANCED
AROMATHERAPY

THE SCIENCE OF ESSENTIAL OIL THERAPY

KURT SCHNAUBELT, PH.D.

Translated from the German by

J. Michael Beasley

Healing Arts Press
Rochester, Vermont

Healing Arts Press
One Park Street
Rochester, Vermont 05767
www.InnerTraditions.com

Healing Arts Press is a division of Inner Traditions International

First U.S. edition published in 1998 by Healing Arts Press
Originally published in German under the title *Neue Aromatherapie by vgs*,
    Cologne, 1995
Copyright © 1995 vgs verlagsgesellschaft, Cologne, Germany
English translation copyright © 1998 Inner Traditions International, Ltd.

Note to the reader: This book is intended as an informational guide. The remedies, approaches, and techniques described herein are meant to supplement, and not to be a substitute for, professional medical care or treatment. They should not be used to treat a serious ailment without prior consultation with a qualified health care professional.

Library of Congress Cataloging-in-Publication Data
Schnaubelt, Kurt.
    [Neue Aromatherapie.   English]
    Advanced aromatherapy : the science of essential oil therapy / Kurt Schnaubelt ;
translated from the German by J. Michael Beasley. — 1st U.S. ed.
        p.   cm.
    Includes bibliographical references and index.
    ISBN 0-89281-743-7 (pbk.)
    1. Aromatherapy.   I. Title.
RM666.A68S36513   1998   97-44453
615'.321—dc21 CIP

Printed and bound in Canada

10 9 8 7 6 5 4

Text design and layout by Kristin Camp
This book was typeset in Goudy with Gill Sans as the display typeface

CONTENTS

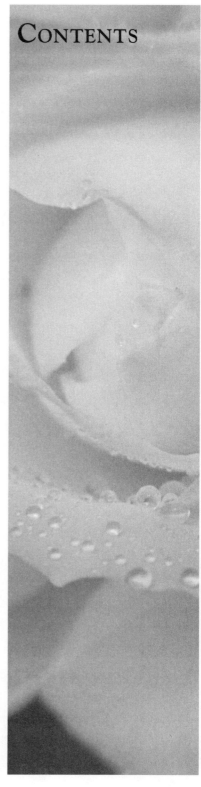

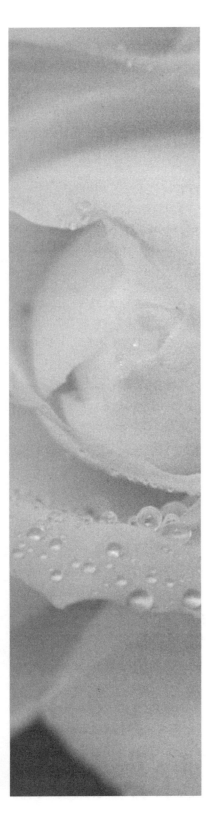

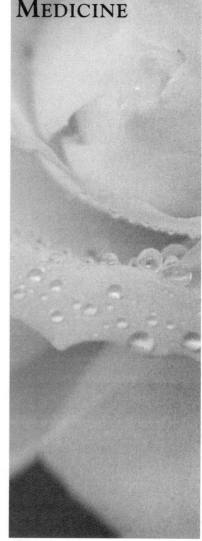

CHAPTER 1

AROMATHERAPY: A CHALLENGE TO CONVENTIONAL MEDICINE

With the end of the millennium upon us, it seems an appropriate time to reflect upon the future of health care. The relevant institutions, at least in Western industrialized societies, are in the midst of an endless and agonizing struggle over the distribution of available funds. Health care is too costly, and trust in the competence and wisdom of the representatives of the health-care system—namely doctors, pharmaceutical companies, equipment manufacturers, and insurance companies—is plummeting. Few people today truly have confidence in conventional health care and medical science. But many who have been hospitalized with a serious illness for any length of time have had to find out the hard way how it feels to be transformed from a patient in need of healing into a helpless victim of an overpowering medical machine. Very few are equipped to withstand the workings of this machine-like institution once they are pulled into its endless maze of treatments, examinations, and subsequent complications.

The existing system has not collapsed entirely because institutions of this size do not simply dissolve into thin air. They are tenacious. It is not consumer confidence but rather monetary magnitude that explains the dominance of this institution and the resulting ability to affect the behavior of society through legislative influence and to affect consciousness and our belief systems by manipulating the direction of science.

Economic considerations leave no doubt that the costs of overpriced treatment methods (which frighten patients with cold technology), medical equipment, and the extremely hierarchical compensation awarded doctors must come down.

Laypeople know instinctively that gyrations of doctors and skirmishes in legislative committees have nothing to do with a patient's health, but everything to do with the distribution of available health-care dollars.

In the long term, no amount of advertising and propaganda will assuage the skepticism of the consumer. Unsettled and disturbed, people turn to alternative methods of health care that replace competition with understanding and compassion and see the patient as a whole person. As these alternative methods turn out to be wholly or partly effective, it becomes obvious just how overpriced the services of conventional medicine are.

Because of its enormous size, the health-care system is finding it difficult to react quickly to the changing needs of its patients. The future of health care lies in fields such as aromatherapy, acupuncture, herbal medicine, and homeopathy which the consumer finds attractive.

The competitive advantages of aromatherapy are apparent. Used in conjunction with other alternative healing modalities—such as acupuncture—it is sure to become one of the strongest challenges to conventional medicine. One of the reasons for aromatherapy's success is its holistic approach, as compared to the symptom-oriented approach of conventional medicine. At the same time, aromatherapy can be used with an allopathic approach, often having very specific medical effects quite similar to those of conventional medicine. Liberation from a painful bladder infection with essential oils triggers further experimentation for successes with aromatherapy. The immediacy of essential oils initiates a deeper involvement with natural healing for anyone who experiments with it. Aromatherapy indeed offers quick and easy solutions for a broad variety of everyday health problems. With information, careful experimentation, and responsible use of the holistic approach, healing with plants becomes a reality. Otherwise, the conventional alternative is sufficiently known—visits to the doctor, lab tests, antibiotics, yeast infections, antimycotics, and so on in an endless vicious circle.

But aromatherapy would not be so attractive if the only thing it offered was a number of quick, simple, and economical solutions. Anyone who uses essential oils once will continue to explore them and will discover the diverse aspects of natural, aromatic essences—relaxation, stress reduction, immune strengthening, preventive cures, personal hygiene, and other steps on the way to healing and staying healthy.

In addition, the aspect of scent cannot be overestimated. Aromatherapy activates the olfactory process and lets us rediscover the nearly forgotten aromas of plants. Perhaps aroma-therapy's greatest asset lies in its ability to demonstrate the link between physical and emotional health to the user. Over time, what develops is an intuitive understanding of how natural scents, their medicinal application, and their influence on emotional well-being combine to form a healing network that far surpasses the mere counteracting of symptoms offered by conventional medicine.

The methodical principle of science is to explain observed effects as direct consequences of clearly identifiable causes. Applied to natural substances, such as essential oils, this principle implies a reduction of the observed effects to one or more "active" ingredients. In the case of German chamomile (*Matricaria recutita*), for example, it was demonstrated that the chamazulene and (–)α-bisabolol were the compounds responsible for its anti-inflammatory effects. The problem does not lie in the method itself, but in the consequences that result when this method becomes dogma and is applied to phenomena for which it is simply not suited or when more appropriate means of viewing natural phenomena are prohibited. Lavender oil, for instance, is seldom used to treat burns in conventional settings because its effectiveness cannot be linked to one or two "active" ingredients (which could be extracted and patented). As a result, there is no financial incentive to research the complex effects of lavender oil.

An expression of this arrogance can be seen in the detrimental effects of antibiotic use on which established pharmacological wisdom—in a mixture of economic power and reductionism elevated to dogma—continues to insist. To avoid misunderstandings, it should be stated that the reductionist method can be a useful tool. It is the institutionalization of reductionism to the exclusion of all other methods which leads to a limited way of perceiving reality.

Antibiotics: The Downfall of Conventional Medicine

The results of reductionism confront us wherever we look. The clearest example is the consequences of antibiotic use—especially among infants and children—which are openly discussed even by conventional physicians. Negative side-effects of antibiotic use are well known and the typical attitude regarding this issue can be summarized as follows: *Prescribe antibiotics only when absolutely necessary.*

In practice, this means that a few rare cases in which antibiotics have been a life-saving measure serve to sell a method of treatment that otherwise may be inappropriate or even harmful to our health. In fact, the phrase "only when absolutely necessary" implies that antibiotics are the most effective treatment available. But that is simply not true, because, prescribed too early and too often, antibiotics weaken the body's immune status.

After spectacular successes during World War II and in the science-crazed 1950s, sulfa-drugs and antibiotics became immensely popular. Naturally, pharmaceutical companies wanted to perpetuate this situation. As a result, and despite all warnings to the contrary, antibiotics are still recklessly overprescribed, often for conditions for which they are ineffective, such as viral illnesses.

Some of the problems caused by overuse of antibiotics include:[1]

1. Antibiotics should help to *defend* against infections. Since they are the cause of resistant germs, however, they *create* chronic infections.
2. The appearance of antibiotic-resistant bacteria has exceeded crisis proportions and can only be described as a growing catastrophe.
3. Many bacteria that cause infections of the respiratory tract, skin, bladder, and

large intestine are resistant to all common antibiotics.[2]

4. The random elimination of beneficial bacteria by antibiotics gives opportunistic organisms such as *Candida albicans* (a ubiquitous yeast fungus) free reign to spread. Metabolic waste products of candida consequently inhibit the efficient functioning of the immune system.

5. Antibiotics suppress the immune response, drastically increasing the chances of recurring infections, as compared to cases treated without antibiotics.

6. Antibiotics given to young children from birth to age two can lead to the onset of asthma beginning at about age six.

7. Reviewing the available literature leads to the conclusion that widespread antibiotic use is responsible for many "civilization diseases."[3] One example is chronic fatigue syndrome (CFS): up to 80 percent of patients diagnosed with CFS have a history of repeated antibiotic use.[4]

Civilization from One Source

Bleak developments are not limited to the pharmaceutical field but are also surfacing in the food industry. According to Eugene P. Grisanti, the CEO of IFF, a leading flavor and fragrance company in New York, the proportion of *artificial* flavor and fragrance materials will increase rapidly,

because modern man wants to eat healthy *and* fast. As consumers demand healthier food choices, it becomes necessary to remove the undesired components such as salt, fat, and cholesterol from the foods. But since the fatty parts of foods contain desirable flavors and aromas, once they are removed they must be replaced with artificial flavors. In addition, taking out fat and cholesterol also leads to a loss of texture and consistency, making it necessary to restore it with artificial consistency agents. Grisanti also pointed out that international variations of the regulation of food purity present undesirable hindrances to the spread of this "brave new world" of flavors. Such impediments, he suggests, should be lifted as soon as possible to allow the consumer quick and easy access to these "wonderful, new taste sensations."

The question then arises: Who is served by these developments? Is it the customer, as is often claimed, or the manufacturers and retailers of these goods? The answer should be obvious: Even the staunchest proponents of free-market economy predict that the manufacture and consumption of an unnecessary diversity of consumer goods has a limited future, since products of the mass market increasingly serve the needs of the producers, and not the consumers.[5]

Betrayed and helpless, we are at the mercy of the powers that be when all of life's needs are provided by one single source. We sense the cynicism, but see the truth only reluctantly in a vain attempt to protect our worldview from grim reality. In fact, cynicism is even more pervasive than generally feared. Not only do big financial institutions own shares in fragrance and food companies, they also hold interest in firms producing pesticides linked to causing breast cancer[6] and at the same time rake in profits from the medications used to treat it. The scientific and economic necessities are staggering and diversity has been all but eliminated so as not to get in the way of business. More and more, our lives are determined by the one-dimensionality of synthetic chemical products. It is difficult to clarify how profitable this system of reductionism really is. One definite result, however, is the reduction of experiences and information that we take in, and the real loss of our relationship to nature.

Where we once turned to the naturally diverse substances found in an herbal tea, today we take a pill with one, two, or three active ingredients. Where we once enjoyed the taste of real strawberries in real yogurt, today we find the penetrating aroma of standardized, artificial fruit flavors along with the guar-gum consistency agent in homogenized, fat-free yogurt.

This massive processing and standardization of our foods should alarm consumers, not the least because these "new" and "wonderful" synthetic fragrances and additives are not substances to which the human body has been acclimated to over a long period of evolution. Many of these new substances are completely synthetic and, like antibiotics and pesticides, contribute to overloading our system with chemicals that heavily tax our organs of metabolism and elimination. The body responds to the chemical overload by inventing "civilization diseases" such as neurodermatitis or CFS.

Aromatherapy: An Answer

It is no accident that aromatherapy has developed in response to these trends. We live in an age when the individual, depending on place of residence, experience, or social status, is faced—in varying degrees—with the effects of our high-tech civilization and the consequences of scientific reductionism. The loss of nature is equally painful for rich and poor. Increased ecological awareness has led to the renewal of "green zones" and to the protection of forests, lakes, and mountains. Those who can flee to those regions of the globe still untouched by the devastation of techno-civilization. Regardless of how the conflicts over ecological questions will be resolved, the fact remains that the majority of people today suffer from the loss of nature. The desire for more nature and less technology is often expressed in vague or ill-defined ways. The ambiguous language of many aromatherapy books, the move toward esotericism that can be found in many of those works, and the conscious departure from the (pseudo-)precise language of medicine and pharmacology are all indicative of this phenomenon.

Aromatherapy can be a first step in overcoming separation of mind and emotion, of body and soul. The esoteric trend in contemporary aromatherapy literature may be a sign of the attempt to bridge this gap. Aromatherapy thereby mirrors a fundamental cultural trend. Theodore Roszak[7] proclaims the end of Freudian psychology in which the soul is an autonomous, scientifically curable entity. According to Roszak, psychology will only have a chance when it takes into account more than just human beings but also nature and the planet on which we live. Likewise, new research in the area of neuropsychology points in the same direction, showing the relationship between emotions, healing, and health.[8] The search for ways to overcome the alienation caused by techno-civilization is a widespread phenomenon not limited to the realm of aromatherapy.

What is impressive about aromatherapy is that it allows us to overcome part of this alienation so easily. In the bottle of essential oil that we bring home from the natural food store, we find more than a lavender or a rosemary oil. We find the fragrances of Provence, smells that elicit memories of our grandmother's clothes chest, but they are also a practical way to relieve the itch of a mosquito bite, saving us from incessant scratching and bleeding. In unifying these disparate elements, we intuitively feel the impact of reductionism fading. For those stressed by civilization, aromatherapy offers nature in a bottle. Nature interacting with humans in many more ways than are possible for conventional products.

The Immune System: Not a One-Way Street

It is safe to assume that the human body will tolerate substances with which it has evolved for millennia far better than substances such as DDT or dioxin. With these obviously toxic substances the case is clear. But is the same not true for other substances that officially are not considered toxic, such as dyes, fragrances, and food additives? It is not very bold to suggest that these substances, which are equally foreign to the human body, also put a strain on our natural defenses.

The conventional models and systems for measuring toxicity are not sensitive enough, and are too reductionistic to accurately assess the many possible ways in which the human ecosystem is thrown out of balance. How else can it be

explained that substances known to cause allergic reactions, toxic shock, emotional imbalance, and a number of other serious problems are routinely added to our foods?

It may be not only the obvious or hidden toxicity in our medications and foods but also the one-dimensionality, the loss of diversity (in life), that weakens the immune system. It will be a long time before science admits that the human immune system functions best when external stimuli are complex and varied. Nonetheless, laypeople have made these connections intuitively and have learned to act accordingly: Getting fresh air, a change of scenery, taking vacations—all the things which we associate with health and well-being and that help firm up the body's complex natural processes. In our technology-driven lives, our innate ability to gather experience is impoverished through processed, one-dimensional products like artificial crab meat, mass-produced wine, PSE (pale, soft, and exuded) pork, hormone-fed chicken, mass-produced furniture with synthetic veneers, as well as digital music and computer-manipulated images on the TV screen. The loss of diverse stimuli is as present as the one-dimensional substitutes. The most recent culmination of this is "virtual reality," in which the simplified substitute has become a total victory over the original. In the realm of health and well-being, aromatherapy fulfills the urge to leave the world of mass markets behind.

Complex Information from Plants

Genuine essential oils—as they are encountered upon distillation—are distinguished by a remarkable diversity of complex substances the likes of which only nature can produce.[9] Like the colored pieces of glass in a kaleidoscope, essential oils are made up of an ever-changing mélange of active main ingredients, secondary components, and trace compounds which lend oils their scents. The composition of essential oils depends upon many factors, such as growing conditions, climate, methods of harvesting, and distillation.

If these oils are not standardized, they offer an inexhaustible reservoir of diversity and are the best way to provide modern man with a pleasant, safe, effective, and accessible means to utilize the pharmacologically active ingredients found in plants. Due to their complexity, genuine essential oils have achieved results that their mass-produced, standardized, watered-down namesakes can never hope to equal.

This complexity, along with the desire for a holistic approach, has brought about a renewed interest in aromatherapy. The risks associated with the use of genuine essential oils are minimal, especially when compared to the much greater risks associated with conventional medicine.

Aromatherapy invites us to experiment and to experience and—above all—it offers us the opportunity to assume more responsibility for our own health and well-being.

The History of Aromatherapy

Originally, the oils produced for the flavor and fragrance industries were the only ones available for the practice of aromatherapy. Such oils were routinely standardized, diluted, or otherwise treated with the goal of meeting the industrial user's needs, which is uniform quality at the lowest possible price. This "doctoring" of essential oils was not carried out with deceitful intentions but was a response to the needs of the fragrance industry. Standardization is not only desirable for the fragrance industry, but it is actually required by certain pharmaceutical manuals which set standards for minimum concentrations of active ingredients, unfortunately, with no criteria for purity.

The criteria established by the pharmaceutical manuals are misleading for the purposes of aromatherapy. How many of us have come to assume a certain standard of quality and purity when we see the abbreviation U.S.P. (United States Pharmacopoeia)? Nevertheless, with pharmaceutical grade, quality is definitely not what we are getting. These manuals only state the minimum concentrations required of certain substances; it makes no difference if these substances are of natural origin or not. Even worse, if these should happen to be synthetic materials, the pharmaceutical manual is ominously silent where impurities or by-products are concerned. Entries appearing under the heading of essential oils in the pharmacopoeias are from another age, when what was good for the manufacturer had to be good for the consumer.

In René-Maurice Gattefossé's original work,[10] a reductionist conviction was conveyed with no critical distance: Active ingredients in the oils should be enriched and less desirable components removed. To insure the effects of the oils, minimum concentrations of active ingredients were proposed.

For decades, Gattefossé's book found few interested readers. Only in 1964, when Dr. Jean

Valnet published his book, did aromatherapy become more widely known.[11] Gattefossé made aromatherapy into a discipline whereas Valnet's work led to its increasing popularity. But even Valnet still reflects the reductionist spirit of his time as there is a clear emphasis on the pharmacologically known components.

In 1978 Paul Belaiche published his three-volume study on the clinical uses of aromatherapy for treating a wide range of infectious and degenerative illnesses.[12] As a result, aromatherapy began to achieve a certain level of acceptance by conventional doctors in France, and insurance companies even paid for treatments. As aromatherapy slowly gained acceptance by conventional medicine, Henri Viaud made new demands for the purity of essential oils. Viaud, a highly important pioneer of French aromatherapy, catalogued the conditions which essential oils had to fulfill to be fit for medicinal use. He also introduced the basic terminology: Oils for medicinal purposes should be *genuine* (absolutely unchanged through any type of manipulation) and *authentic* (only the oil from a specific type of plant). In retrospect, it is clear that the greatest advance made in the development of aromatherapy was the return to genuine oils derived exclusively from one species of plant. Only then did some producers in France begin to manufacture oils according to these requirements. This was the birth of modern aromatherapy.

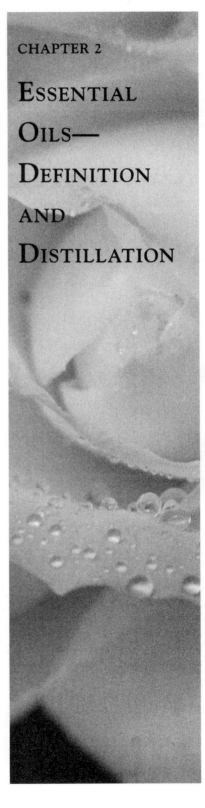

Plant Messengers

Essential oils play very important and diverse roles in plant metabolism. They serve to attract beneficial insects and defend against harmful microorganisms. Moreover, essential oils allow plants to send and receive signals and to communicate with one another.

It is probable that the simultaneous evolution of plants and plant-eaters led to the development of a chemical system of communication. Nutritional elements attracted plant-eaters of both sexes, resulting in the meeting of potential sexual partners at feeding places. Animals imitate the attracting plant signals by releasing similar scents, to attract a mate, for example. This is a simple communication system based on "borrowed" chemical messages.[1]

Chemical Messages

Chemical communication requires specific signals that can be clearly recognized and interpreted. They must be distinguishable from "background scents" that are naturally present in the environment. Normally this is achieved through a unique, multifaceted mixture of less specified molecules. In nature, we often observe synergistic effects of multiple components in a "bouquet" of chemical messengers. Nature prefers this solution to the complex synthesis of substances having specific, narrow functions. For example, the attracting pheromone for the bark beetle consists of an acetal and an ester. Pure acetal alone has very little activity, pure ester even less, but their combination is highly active. The specific acetal is not unique to the bark beetle. It has been identified in the scents of various plants. The ester has been identified in the secretions of another beetle and the scent of the Bartlett pear.

The effectiveness of chemical messengers hinges on another important factor, the symmetry of their molecular structure: organic molecules can consist of identical atoms but have different configurations in space. Two such molecules—which are mirror images of each other (something like a right and a left glove)—are called enantiomers.

Bark beetles, for example, use terpenes for chemical communication and create predominantly or exclusively one enantiomer. They are able to create an enantiomer ratio specific to their species which would lose its effectiveness if altered even slightly: it would no longer be recognized by other bark beetles.

One example from the plant world is the terpene alcohol α-bisabolol, which can be found in two enantiomeric forms, $(+)\alpha$-bisabolol and $(-)\alpha$-bisabolol. In the essential oil of German chamomile mainly the effective $(-)\alpha$-bisabolol is encountered. The chemical synthesis of α-bisabolol, however, yields a 50:50 racemic mixture of $(+)\alpha$-bisabolol and $(-)\alpha$-bisabolol. Synthetic bisabolol, known as levomenol, is therefore not called bisabolol but racemic bisabolol.

It is interesting to note how much humans have been able to learn about insects, and how little of this knowledge we are willing to apply to the use of essential oils. Having examined how wonderfully precisely nature communicates with the help of terpenes (see pages 23–24), and how the natural compositions guarantee uniqueness, we should realize that natural essential oils work more extensively and effectively than watered-down, synthetic imitations from the kegs of the fragrance industry.

The reductionist style of treating essential oils as just another group of chemicals ignores the fact that not only beetles and plants have developed together, but also humans and plants. The interaction between humans and plants, and consequently between humans and natural essential oils, proved to be so successful and valuable that humans cultivated specific plants, especially kitchen herbs, contributing to the survival of these species.

Analyses show that essential oils primarily consist of terpenes, terpene-related compounds, and phenylpropane derivates. We find among the terpenes all varieties of messengers, from sex attractants to highly effective defense signals. It helps to keep the information character of these aromatic molecules of the animal and plant world in mind as we look at the effects of essential oils on the healing process.

Essential Oils—Distillation, Chemistry, and History

The ISO (International Organization for Standardization) Vocabulary of Natural Materials

(ISO/DIS 9235.2)[2] defines an essential oil as follows:

> An essential oil is a product made by distillation with either water or steam or by mechanical processing of citrus rinds or by dry distillation of natural materials. Following the distillation, the essential oil is physically separated from the water phase.

In the broadest sense, essential oils are produced by steam distillation. Through the process of distillation the oily components of the plant are separated from the watery ones. Distillation is a very old process and has been practiced, in one form or another, in many cultures. Because the process is familiar, we assume that the distillation of essential oils is a natural process. But this is only true insofar as the main agent of the process is life-giving water. Otherwise, steam distillation is a technical process, and the composition of plant constituents that we produce this way is to some degree arbitrary, depending on plant and distillation conditions.

These oily, volatile components are the basis of plant scents. They are either end products or by-products of plant metabolism, and are stored in the plants in special organs. Through steam distillation these essential oils are extracted from these special glands or ducts in a complex physical-chemical process.

Steam Distillation

The technical aspects of extracting essential oils have been described in detail elsewhere (Günther,[3] Gildemeister,[4] Denny[5]), so they shall only be reiterated briefly here.

Essential oils are extracted from natural raw materials through water or steam distillation. Its basic principles are illustrated in the diagram on page 12. Plant material is heated with water and brought to a boil. The steam containing the volatile essential oil is run through a cooler, where it condenses, and the liquid distillate is gathered. The essential oil appears as a thin film on top of the liquid. In few cases, the oil is heavier than water and sinks to the bottom. Through special technical processes, the oil is separated from the water.

Those components of the plant that are volatile but also water soluble—among them valuable and useful substances—will not separate but remain dissolved in water. Therefore, the distillation water, the aromatic hydrosol, is often used in aromatherapy, because these water-soluble aromatic substances are usually more mild and less irritating than those found in the essential oils themselves and have their own beneficial effects.

Essential oils do not exist in plants as free-moving substances but are stored in microscopic cellular containers. The steam generated in the steam distillation process frees the oils and binds with some substances while splitting others, thus creating new compounds (chamazulene—a blue-tinted hydrocarbon, for example, does not exist in the same form in the plant). These processes normally are not considered in the physicochemical descriptions of essential oil distillation.

If we survey the various methods of distillation and the various types of oils they produce, it becomes clear that distillation is just as much an art as it is a science. Such factors as cultivation and harvesting, methods of preparing materials for distillation, special characteristics of the

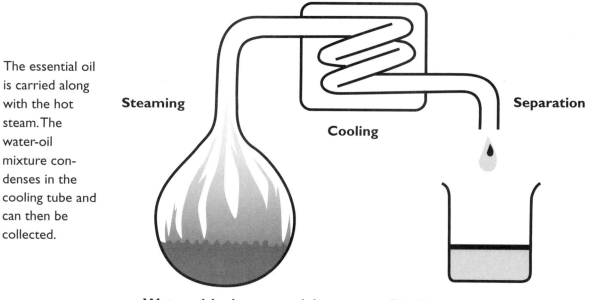

The essential oil is carried along with the hot steam. The water-oil mixture condenses in the cooling tube and can then be collected.

Steaming

Cooling

Separation

Water with plant material

Distilled water and essential oil

equipment used, the duration of the distillation process, and many others all influence the final product. An essential oil is not simply the calculated product of a precisely quantifiable physicochemical process, but the product of the person making it.

The entire process, from gathering plants to distillation, ideally should be performed by the same person and the producer should see his product as a result of complex factors and created for the special needs of aromatherapy. A number of factors— the skill of the distiller, growing region, climate, and variations in cultivation and harvesting—will influence the quality and character of the finished oil. Distilling essential oils is more closely related to producing a fine wine than to making a standardized fragrance: both are dependent upon the interplay between man and nature. Production of essential oils should require—as is typical in the wine trade—that es-

sential oils intended for use in aromatherapy are traded with a clear designation of the producer.

Conditions particular to the distillation process produce some useful results for aromatherapy. Oils made by steam distillation inevitably contain materials that are inert when exposed to water, which means they react very little or not at all. For this reason, other comparatively subtle effects come into play, which are based on the lipophilic nature of the molecules. Hydrophilic molecules remain dissolved in the water and are difficult to separate.

The physical nature of essential oils—a low molecular weight combined with pronounced lipophilic tendencies—allows them to penetrate human tissue more quickly than any other substance.[6] This is what gives aromatherapy its effectiveness.

Essential oils are the products of plant metabolism. Each plant has a particular organ for

Modern Extraction Processes

Naturally, producers in the age of modern technology have not limited themselves to the traditional methods of producing oils. They have developed new, gentler, and higher-yielding variations of classic distillation methods, such as hydrodiffusion, in which the steam runs through the plant material from top to bottom.

Carbon dioxide extraction

Some entirely new methods have been developed as well. The most significant is carbon dioxide extraction. This process exploits the ability of carbon dioxide to transform into a special aggregate state, which the physicist calls supercritical. In this state carbon dioxide exhibits qualities of both a gas and a liquid.

For this type of extraction, the gas must be under high pressure at a constant temperature (approximately 30°C), and the required equipment is very expensive. The process runs at much lower temperatures than steam distillation, and is therefore more gentle. The aromas of oils derived from this process are astoundingly true to those of the plant, and the extracts are very pure since the oils come into contact with only the carbon dioxide. Unfortunately, the complexity and costs involved in CO_2 extraction make these oils relatively expensive. For this reason, CO_2 extraction is usually limited to producing only expensive herbal or floral oils.

Phytonic process

The phytonic process provides an even gentler method of extraction than carbon dioxide extraction. Developed in England, this process extracts the oils at even lower temperatures (room temperature or lower) than CO_2 extraction, using new agents that are bashfully called "non-CFCs" (non-chlorofluorocarbons).

Oils extracted by this method (named "phytols" by the inventor) are perhaps as close to their natural form as possible. While the process does not use ozone-depleting CFCs, it does use fluorocarbons (or correctly fluorohydrocarbons) which are also potentially harmful and do not seem adequate for heightened ecological consciousness.

producing or storing an oil, for example, the glandular hairs in the outer cell layer (epidermis) of the labiate varieties (Lamiaceae) such as thyme, marjoram, savory, rosemary, and sage. These oil (or hair) cells are living cells filled with essential oils or resin. We find oil cells in the laurel (Lauraceae) family, such as cinnamon. Essential oils, resins, or balsams can be found in the oil and hair canals, and cavities of plant tissue. Often, as the neighboring cells recede, the cavities expand and become tubelike. Cavities of this type are found in plants of the Umbelliferae family, such as anise, caraway, fennel, coriander, and celery. If these plants are damaged or cut, considerable amounts of resin are produced in the plant tissue. True oil "containers" are formed when the cell walls of the oil-producing cells dissolve, and the resulting cavity becomes the container for the oil. This type of oil container can be found in citrus rinds.

Essential oils can be produced in any part of

the plant: In rose and jasmine, essential oils are produced in the flowers; in geranium, patchouli, and peppermint they are produced in the leaves; in anise and nutmeg they are produced in the fruit; in celery, cardamom, and parsley, in the seeds; in lemon and orange, in the rinds; in angelica and vetiver, in the roots; and in sandalwood and cedar they are produced in the wood. Essential oils are also found in herbs and grasses such as tarragon, thyme, lemongrass, and citronella, in the needles and branches of pine, spruce, fir, and cypress, and in the resin and balsam of galbanum, myrrh, and frankincense, or in the bark of cinnamon. Some plants, like the bitter orange tree, produce oils with different compositions in different parts of the plant. The flowers of bitter orange produce neroli oil, the leaves produce petitgrain oil, and the rinds of the fruit produce bitter orange oil.

Essential Oil Terminology

The composition of essential oils used for therapeutic purposes is of critical importance. It is clear that two oils of differing chemical compositions will have markedly different pharmacological and healing effects. This simple fact has been long ignored by medical science. Examination of published studies on the therapeutic effects of essential oils reveals that these studies have not paid much attention to the significance of the chemical makeup of these essential oils.

It is a mystery why modern research, which normally scrutinizes even the smallest details, has studied essential oils without giving due attention to their chemical compositions. No wonder various studies of the same oil often would have con-

tradictory results. Such studies would frequently report on oils of the same name but different chemical makeups. Defining and describing oils precisely is crucial, and a trend in this direction began in the late 1970s. In order to accurately analyze the chemical composition of an essential oil, it is necessary to distill it from only one plant variety, even though the ratios of individual components may vary due to climatic influences, growing region, and time of harvest.

Correct Botanical Descriptions: Chamomile Is Not Always Chamomile

For many oils, it is not always possible to clearly identify the plant source by its common name, such as eucalyptus or chamomile.

We know, for example, that there are hundreds of different eucalyptus varieties throughout the world, each producing a different essential oil. The oils from the leaves of *Eucalyptus globulus*, for example, differ significantly from the oils distilled from *Eucalyptus radiata*. These differ substantially from the oils of *Eucalyptus dives* and *Eucalyptus citriodora*.

Each of these varieties differs in chemical composition, which in turn results in different uses for aromatherapy. The high terpene alcohol (see page 25) content of *Eucalyptus radiata* renders it an excellent antiviral agent used in aromatherapy for conditions of the upper respiratory tract. On the other hand, *Eucalyptus dives*, thanks to its ketone content (see page 27), is valued—especially when combined with *Eucalyptus radiata*—as a mucolytic. *Eucalyptus citriodora* contains aldehydes (see page 27), such as citral and citronellal, and is a reliable sedative. These examples illustrate the importance of using the correct botanical designation for its appropriate use in aromatherapy.

The situation is similar with chamomile. The oils of several different plants are known by this name, but only some of them are actually distilled from a genuine chamomile. There are oils that contain a blue hydrocarbon (azulene) which lends them a color similar to that of chamomile. Occasionally they are sold under the name of chamomile, but they are actually distilled from a relative of wormwood, namely *Artemisia arborescens*. While the oil of German chamomile (*Matricaria recutita*) is safe, oils from the mugwort family, which are occasionally sold as chamomile, are toxic due to the presence of thujone, which can lead to damage of the central nervous system, epileptic seizures, or liver damage.

There are also some major differences between the two main types of chamomile, German chamomile and Roman chamomile: the blue German chamomile oil contains chamazulene, which has strong anti-inflammatory effects, while Roman chamomile oil is primarily an antispasmodic.

Chemotypes

As a rule, chemical composition is consistent among different plants of the same botanical species, but there are some occasional differences. The most important examples of this are rosemary and thyme. The chemical composition of rosemary varies greatly according to whether the plant is grown inland or near the coast. Apart from the factors of growing region and climate, this phenomenon has never been fully explained. For our purposes, it is sufficient only to acknowledge that it does occur.

This is known in the scientific literature as chemical polymorphism. In such cases, the bo-

tanical name along with the name of the characteristic component is used. These are chemical "races," or chemotypes.[7]

There are three distinct chemotypes of rosemary: the oils from Spain or the former Yugoslavia contain a relatively high amount of camphor, or borneol, so we call this chemotype *borneol type*; the oils from Africa, distinguished by a high cineole content, are called *cineole type*; and the oils from the south of France or Corsica, especially rich in verbenone, are called *verbenone type*.

Consequently, varying compositions make each oil suitable for different uses in aromatherapy. The borneol type is especially suited for stimulating elimination from the liver and kidneys and for relaxing tense muscles; the cineole type is best used for catarrhal infections; and the verbenone type, because of its regenerative qualities, is best suited for skin care.

Thymus vulgaris, the herb that we know as thyme, is another labiate in which we can see pronounced polymorphism. There are at least seven different chemotypes of thyme, each with its own unique chemical composition. They are primarily distinguished by their phenol content (see page 24). There are thyme chemotypes with a strong thymol[8] and/or carvacrol content, and there are additional types with high percentages of terpene alcohols such as linalol, geraniol, or thujanol. The linalol and thujanol chemotypes are used most frequently in aromatherapy.

Quality Control

The successful practice of aromatherapy demands the use of genuine essential oils and the consistent control of their quality and purity.

A look at the development of aromatherapy

should really begin with the books by Valnet and Tisserand. At the time these were written, demand for essential oils intended exclusively for aromatherapy was minimal. Aromatherapy practitioners found essential oils through established importers who gathered extracts from all corners of the globe sold primarily to the flavor and fragrance trade. Naturally, producers provided what their customers needed. Genuine oils as understood in aromatherapy were not produced; rather, the oils produced were those that were—as was customary—adjusted to the requirements of their industrial users. From the discrepancy between what was needed in aromatherapy and what was available, a great deal of confusion, misunderstanding, and disappointment resulted.

So it was up to those who used essential oils for therapeutic purposes to establish their own criteria for purity and genuineness of essential oils. Even for the aromatherapy enthusiast who is only marginally interested in science, it is therefore important to have at least a basic understanding of the current possibilities for analyzing the composition of essential oils.

In 1979 Kubeczka[9] developed guidelines for determining the quality of essential oils used for medicinal purposes. According to Kubeczka, the pharmaceutical effects of essential oils are based on the presence of chemical components that complement each other in a synergistic way. Determining the *concentration* of a specific component in an oil (such as cineole in eucalyptus oil, for example) is absolutely insufficient for determining the *quality* of a particular essential oil. Otherwise a synthetic oil would be just as effective as a natural essential oil.

Methods of Standardization

As already mentioned, various pharmacopoeias defined the quality of an oil by prescribing a minimum content of a certain "active" ingredient. Consequently, processors would add the value-giving component if its concentration was not sufficient, for example, the ester linalyl acetate in lavender oil. It is often relatively simple to recognize, by means of chemical analysis, when synthetic materials have been added to a natural product, as impurities, which are originally not present in the oil, are brought into the natural substance along with the synthetic one. These impurities can serve as an indicator for doctoring. As analytical methods became more refined, so did the methods of adulteration. Insiders report instances when, for example, linalyl acetate was sprayed on lavender plants just before harvest to guarantee a sufficient concentration in the distilled oil without having to add the substance in a "fraudulent manner" to the finished oil.

Another type of "cutting" is widely established—the more or less complete reconstruction of essential oils, in which the main components of an oil are simply mixed together. Often the substances used in this process are of natural origin so that the finished product can justifiably be called "natural." The fragrance of these oils is often weak and insipid, but it can be intensified by adding small quantities of true natural oils or synthetic fragrances.

Well-known French distillers have confirmed that such practices are widespread in the fragrance industry. They estimate that, in this fashion, from one liter of pure distilled rosemary oil, for example, twenty liters will result to be sold to retailers.

The accessibility of improved analytical methods for retailers and users of essential oils can lead only to the availability of higher quality oils. Informed buying and demand for higher quality oils will bypass makers of watered-down, doctored oils. More and more businesses specializing in aromatherapy now buy from producers who make their oils according to the stringent demands of aromatherapy, and not for the perfume and fragrance industry.

Without a doubt, genuine oils are much more expensive than adulterated oils. If one has spent some time working with genuine oils, the nose is often (though regrettably not always) a reliable partner in distinguishing between genuine oils and their synthetic counterparts. But keep in mind that the most expensive oils are also the most potent, and therefore the most cost-effective: they require the smallest amounts to achieve their effects.

It would be desirable if aromatherapy purveyors took advantage of analytical tools, and brought as much clarity as possible to the business. It is consistent with holistic thinking to treat essential oils not just as standardized mixtures of substances (as the pharmacy manuals do) but as complex products of the cooperation between man and nature. Why should a fine bergamot oil from Sicily not be treated like a good bottle of wine, with information on the vintage and its producer provided on the label?

According to Kubeczka, evaluating the quality of an essential oil cannot be restricted to determining its main component, but must take into account trace elements as well. The effect achieved by the interaction of a variety of components has a different quality than simply adding together individual effects. Putting it simply, the effects of the whole are greater than the effects of the sum of its parts.

To analyze the composition of an oil and to determine the quality of an oil require a number of analytical methods. The applied method has to be able to identify and quantify as many components of the oil as possible. Gas chromatography fulfills a large part of these requirements.

Gas chromatography

Gas chromatography is a method of separating volatile compounds. The gaseous (mobile) phase carries the vaporized sample through an absorbent column (stationary phase) in which the individual components separate. When the individual components leave the column, they generate a signal in a detector. In the resulting graphic depiction (chromatogram) the area of a peak is, as a rule, proportional to the amount of the substance causing it, allowing individual concentrations to be determined.

Gas chromatography, then, allows us to separate an essential oil into its individual components. The result of such an analysis is called the chromatogram of the oil. If the chromatograms of two or more oils are the same we can assume that the oils are the same, or at least that they are from the same plant variety.

But gas chromatography does not allow us to identify or name all the components found in an essential oil. Only through long comparative tests of single substances can we determine which individual substances cause the peak on the chromatogram. If the peak of a test substance shows up at the same spot as a peak in the chromatogram it can be assumed that the test substance and the compound in the oil are identical. The correct and meaningful interpretation of a gas chromatogram therefore requires a great deal of expertise.

Mass spectrometry

Nonetheless, such evaluations of essential oils are often unsatisfactory and ambiguous. Modern analytical technology allows us to go a step further and combine gas chromatography with a mass spectrometer, called GC–MS. With this combination of analytical tools, it is possible to separate the components and identify each component precisely according to its molecular mass spectrum. With the help of modern electronic data processing, we can compare the resulting mass spectrograms with those in computer libraries, and thus make an exact identification. Yet sesquiterpene

compounds, which can have very similar mass spectrograms, often still require the experience of the chemist to be clearly differentiated.

One method has been developed recently that allows detection of doctoring of essential oils with natural substances: enantiomer selective gas chromatography. As already described (see pages 9–10), plants have the ability to manufacture oil molecules in very special enantiomeric ratios that are characteristic of each plant. As with bisabolol in German chamomile, borneol found in rosemary oil comes in a very unique ratio of its (+)- and (−)-form, which is different from that of other plants. If natural borneol from cheaper plants is added to rosemary oil, the resulting change in the borneol ratio can be detected.

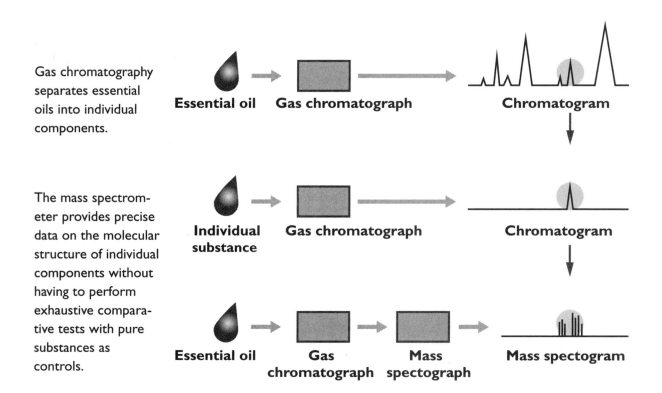

Gas chromatography separates essential oils into individual components.

Essential oil **Gas chromatograph** **Chromatogram**

The mass spectrometer provides precise data on the molecular structure of individual components without having to perform exhaustive comparative tests with pure substances as controls.

Individual substance **Gas chromatograph** **Chromatogram**

Essential oil **Gas chromatograph** **Mass spectograph** **Mass spectogram**

The Composition of Essential Oils

In many seminars at the Pacific Institute of Aromatherapy, it happens that newcomers who are eager to start recording recipes do not want to be bothered with the chemistry, which they consider a distracting nuisance. But when they find out that essential oils can provide quick, safe treatment for a variety of conditions, yet not in the same manner as taking a pill, they become more interested in the how and why and the underlying chemical basis. To satisfy this interest, it is not necessary to study all of organic chemistry, but only to become familiar with the terminology that we inevitably encounter in the literature. Familiarity with relevant chemical terms has distinct advantages. It opens the way to a simple and elegant system of essential oils, dividing them into twelve groups.

A basic knowledge of the chemical qualities of essential oils is the starting point for understanding the healing powers of aromatherapy. With today's detailed knowledge of the composition of essential oils, and the resulting necessity of using oils in their most natural form, aromatherapy appears more interesting than ever in the fifty years since the publication of Gattefossé's book.

An Aroma Chemistry Primer

Organic chemistry is the chemistry of carbon. Carbon has four chemical bonds and can bond with other carbon atoms, to form chains, branching chains, and rings, often forming very complex structures. Chemistry has developed a special notation to depict these structures.

The molecular building blocks, the atoms, are symbolized by the first letter of the Latin name of the corresponding element: C for carbon, O for oxygen, H for hydrogen, and N for nitrogen. Bonds between atoms are shown as a dash.

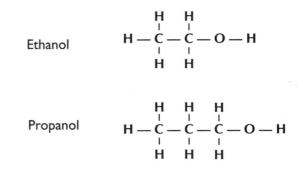

In the case of the terpene molecules, with ten carbon atoms, this notation is already somewhat busy. Here, for example, is the structure of limonene, a monoterpene:

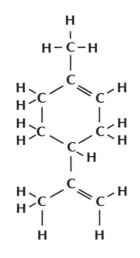

In order to simplify the diagram, the symbols for carbon and hydrogen are omitted and only the geometric structure in which the carbon atoms are linked is shown. The chemical structure for limonene would then look like this:

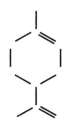

End and corner points of such a structure represent carbon including bonded hydrogen atoms; one dash signifies a single bond, two dashes signify a double bond.

Other elements, such as oxygen or nitrogen, are represented with their chemical symbol and a corresponding chemical bond. The structure of linalol, a monoterpene alcohol, looks like this:

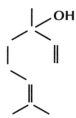

A special ring system is that of benzene. In this case the term "aromatic" comes from the language of chemistry and refers to the ring structure and the special type of bonds between carbon atoms. Bonding energy exceeding that of single bonds is distributed equally over the ring system and is symbolized by a circle inside the six-ring. If a hydrogen atom is replaced by another atom or molecule (R = radical), the remaining structural element is called *phenyl radical.*

Benzene

Phenyl radical

Having the ability to establish four chemical bonds, carbon has nearly limitless possibilities for bonding with other carbon atoms, or other elements, which explains the boundless variety of substances found in so-called organic chemistry. The carbon-carbon chain makes up the backbone of an organic molecule. In typical hydrocarbon molecules, the bonds between two carbon atoms and between carbon and hydrogen atoms are relatively strong. They are nonpolar and, consequently, chemically very stable, so they do not readily react with other molecules.

Functional groups

Oxygen or nitrogen, so-called hetero elements, bring variety to the uniformity of hydrocarbon structures. The bond between carbon and oxygen is polar, which means it has partial positive and negative charges that exert forces on neighboring elements. Therefore, these bonds are chemically more reactive, and most chemical reactions involving these molecules begin at these bonds. Because of this, such structural elements of a molecule—for example, the oxygen-carbon bond—are characterized as functional groups. Especially in smaller molecules, such as the terpenes, the chemical reactivity is determined to a very great extent by the functional group.

Following is a list of the oxygen-containing functional groups which play a significant role in aromatherapy:

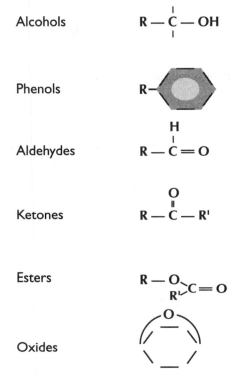

Alcohols	$R - \overset{\mid}{\underset{\mid}{C}} - OH$
Phenols	$R-$
Aldehydes	$R - \overset{H}{\underset{\mid}{C}} = O$
Ketones	$R - \overset{O}{\underset{\parallel}{C}} - R'$
Esters	$R - O \diagdown C = O$
Oxides	

The labels R and R' indicate a site for a bonded structural element or a side chain of multiple carbon atoms.

Main Components of Essential Oils

In order to better understand the effects of essential oils, it is useful to divide their components into two main groups according to their biochemical origin: the terpenes and higher homologues (other molecules based on terpene) on the one hand, and phenylpropane derivatives on the other, which include, among others, cinnamic acid and cinnamic aldehydes. Each of these

groups is created by different biosynthetic processes, which take place in different parts of the plant cells.

By quantity, the terpenes and their higher homologues are the most significant components of essential oils. The backbone of these molecules consists of 10 carbon atoms for monoterpenes, 15 for sesquiterpenes, 20 for diterpenes, and 30 for triterpenes. These molecules are made up of multiples of a basic chemical building block with 5 carbon atoms: isoprene[10] (see figure below). A monoterpene, then, consists of two units of isoprene. The biosynthesis in the plant cell progresses from isoprene with 5 carbon atoms, to molecules with 10 carbon atoms (such as geraniol, a terpene alcohol) and 15 carbon atoms (farnesol, a sesquiterpene alcohol), to larger, more complicated molecules, such as cholesterol, the starting point for the synthesis of other steroids, including important hormones. The relationship of terpenes as the most important active ingredient of essential oils to hormones makes their strong influence on the body more understandable.

$$R - \overset{\mid}{\underset{\mid}{C}} - \overset{\mid}{\underset{\mid}{C}} = C \overset{\diagup C \diagdown}{\underset{\diagdown C \diagup}{}} R'$$

The molecular model for isoprene. R and R' can link to other isoprene molecules, forming long molecular chains.

Phenylpropanes, on the other hand, are by-products of the amino acid metabolism, which is essential for the production of proteins. The breakdown of the amino acid phenyl alanine produces cinnamic acid, which in turn is a building block for such diverse substances as anethol (a component of anise oil), eugenol (a component of clove oil), vanillin (a component of vanilla), or coumarin (a trace component in various oils with strong relaxing effects).

Problems in Classifying Functional Groups

Two chemical families, terpenes and phenylpropanes, make up nearly 100 percent of the components of essential oils. The effects of essential oils can therefore be traced back mostly to the substances in these groups. Gattefossé categorized the components of essential oils according to functional groups: alcohols, aldehydes, ketones, etc. (see pages 20–21), and the development of French aromatherapy is shot through with this concept.

The application of a purely chemical view inevitably led to an overcategorization. As valuable as this concept of categorizing was, it is accurate for only the dominant terpenes. For phenylpropanes, which plants synthesize quite differently, these categories do not apply— even though the functional groups exert their influences here as well. For example, terpene aldehydes have general sedative and anti-inflammatory effects, while cinnamic aldehyde, a phenylpropane, has stimulating and irritating effects.

A modern view takes the biosynthesis of the oil molecules into consideration and offers a consistent system for classifying effects of all the components of essential oils.

Spectrum of Action of Essential Oil Components

The mechanisms of action of essential oils can in a first approximation be explained by twelve important groups of constituents. Oils whose main components belong to the same group will exhibit similar effects. But naturally each oil has its own specific qualities in addition to its general properties. The table on page 23 provides an overview of the most important qualities of monoterpenes, sesquiterpenes, and phenylpropanes.

CLASSIFICATION OF TERPENES AND THEIR NATURAL OCCURENCE

	Number of units of isoprene	Found in
Monoterpenes	2	essential oils
Sesquiterpenes	3	essential oils, bitters, balsams
Diterpenes	4	essential oils, resins, balsams, Vitamin A, gibberellin
Triterpenes	6	resins, sterols, steroids, hormones
Tetraterpenes	8	pigments (such as carotenoids)
Polyterpenes	>8	plant fluids (latex), gutta-percha, rubber

INFLUENCE OF FUNCTIONAL GROUPS ON THE EFFECTS OF ESSENTIAL OIL COMPONENTS

	Molecule type	Effects	Found in
Monoterpenes	Monoterpene-hydrocarbons	stimulant	pine, orange
	Ketones	mucolytic	sage, hyssop
	Aldehydes	calmative	citronella, melissa
	Esters	antispasmodic	lavender, clary sage
	Alcohols	natural tonic	palmarosa, peppermint, coriander
	Phenols	stimulant, irritant	oregano, thyme
	Oxides	expectorant	eucalyptus, tea tree, niaouli
Sesqui-terpenes	Sesquiterpene-hydrocarbons	anti-inflammatory	German chamomile
	Alcohols (and others)	various	sandalwood, vetiver, patchouli
	Lactones	mucolytic	*Inula graveolens,* laurel
Phenyl-propanes	Estragol	antispasmodic	tarragon
	Anethol	antispasmodic	anise
	Eugenol	sensitizing	clove
	Cinnamic aldehyde	antiseptic	cinnamon, cassia

Spectrum of Action of the Phenylpropanes

All phenylpropanes contain an aromatic ring structure just like the phenols. For instance, cinnamic aldehyde (found in cinnamon bark oil and cassia oil) and eugenol (found in clove bud oil and clove leaf oil) are the two members of the group with stimulant and irritant but also strong antiseptic effects. Other important phenylpropanes, such as estragol (also known as methyl chavicol) in basil and tarragon oil, and anethol, which is found in anise oil, are much less aggressive and have a definite stabi-lizing influence on the autonomic nervous system. They also have strong antispasmodic effects, especially (as one might guess from the culinary usage of these oils) in the digestive tract.

Spectrum of Action of the Terpenes

Essential oils contain only monoterpenes (10 carbon atoms) and sesquiterpenes (15 carbon atoms) in notable quantities. Diterpenes (20 carbon atoms) are encountered only in small quantities and only in a few oils, such as sclareol in clary sage oil (*Salvia sclarea*).

ESSENTIAL OILS WITH PHENYL-PROPANES AS A MAIN COMPONENT

Cinnamic aldehyde: cinnamon (*Cinnamomum ceylanicum*), cassia (*Cinnamomum cassia*)

Eugenol: clove bud, clove leaves (*Eugenia caryophyllata*)

Estragol: basil (*Ocimum basilicum*), tarragon (*Artemisia dracunculus*)

Anethol: anise (*Pimpinella anisum*)

Saffrol: sassafras (*Sassafras albidum*), white camphor (*Cinnamomum camphora*)

Myristicin: nutmeg (*Myristica fragrans*)

Apiol: parsley (*Petroselinum sativum*)

The varying molecular size of monoterpenes and terpenoids and their higher homologues has practical implications for aromatherapy. Monoterpenes[11] are so small that their effects are so greatly influenced by the nature of a functional group that they can be categorized accordingly. For example, terpene aldehydes have calming effects, while terpene alcohols are antiseptic and tonic.

This method of classification cannot readily be applied to the larger sesquiterpenes, because here the influence of the functional group is less dramatic. The effects of these molecules are determined as much by their unique molecular structure as by a functional group, and vary significantly from molecule to molecule.

The bulk (approximately 90 percent) of the components of essential oils are monoterpenes and sesquiterpenes. For a listing of the most important characteristics the functional groups lend to the terpene molecules, see the table on page 23. Monoterpenes are the dominant components of citrus and needle oils, as well as oils derived from herbs and spices. Oxygen-containing monoterpenes, such as geraniol, linalol, nerol, and citral or citronellal, are among the most widely distributed natural terpene compounds. We often find that oils consist primarily of monoterpenes and about 10, 15, or 20 percent sesquiterpenes.

A high monoterpene content can often be recognized by looking at an oil. Oils like eucalyptus are mostly clear, mobile (have a low viscosity), and volatile. These properties reflect the small molecular size of the terpene molecules. Oils with a high sesquiterpene content, such as patchouli or sandalwood, have a much higher viscosity. Their color varies from yellow or dark yellow to brown. Because of their lasting aroma and their low volatility, they are often used as fixatives or base notes.

Monoterpene phenols

Phenol itself (see diagram on page 25) does not exist in the plant world. In contrast to the most common phenols found in essential oils, such as thymol and carvacrol, it is a carcinogen. In addition to a hydroxyl group (OH), there is also a short carbon chain attached to the aromatic ring. These natural substances have nothing in common with phenol, which is poisonous and derived from mineral oil. Rather, they are a perfect example of the advantages natural substances hold over synthetic ones. The antiseptic effect of natural thymol is significantly greater than that of synthetic phenol, but thymol is practically nontoxic compared to its synthetic namesake (see page 47).

Essential oils with high concentrations of the monoterpene-phenols thymol and carvacrol are thyme, ajowan, oregano, summer savory, and winter savory (mountain savory).

OH

Phenol
Pure phenol is toxic.

OH

Thymol
Plant-derived phenols, such as thymol, have additional side chains that transform them into nontoxic, effective antiseptics.

Monoterpene alcohols

Monoterpene alcohols share some similarities with phenols. The hydroxyl group is, however, not attached to an aromatic ring system but to a "normal" terpene structure. They are mild and belong to the gentlest and most useful terpene molecules. Often, they are astoundingly effective against microorganisms, but nontoxic to humans. Essential oils containing primarily monoterpene alcohols are therefore especially suitable for everyday use in hygiene and skin care. Oils with a high monoterpene alcohol content are usually distinguished by their pleasant scent and a tonifying effect, especially on the nerves.

Essential oils with a high content of the monoterpene alcohol linalol are coriander, rosewood, petitgrain, and the linalol chemotype of thyme. Neroli and clary sage also contain high levels of linalol.

METABOLISM OF PLANT CELLS

Biosynthesis of terpenes and phenylpropanes follows two different paths in plant cells.

TERPENES:

Monoterpenes (C10)
Classification according to functional group influence.
Relevant groups:
- Monoterpenes (C10)
- C10-alcohols
- C10-phenols
- C10-aldehydes
- C10-ketones
- C10-esters
- C10-oxides

Sesquiterpenes (C15)
Classification according to functional groups only somewhat useful.
Relevant groups:
- Sesquiterpenes (C15)
- C15-ketones
- C15-lactones

Diterpenes

Cholesterin, steroids, hormones

PHENYLPROPANES:

Functional groups are not suitable for characterizing effects.
Relevant groups:
- Estragol, anethol, etc. (relatively mild molecules)
- Cinnamic aldehyde, eugenol (irritant, can cause sensitivity)

ESSENTIAL OILS WITH MONOTERPENE PHENOLS AS MAIN COMPONENTS

Thyme *(Thymus vulgaris)*

Spanish thyme *(Thymus zygis)*

Ajowan *(Carum opticum)*

Oregano *(Origanum vulgaris, O. compactum)*

Summer savory *(Satureja hortensis)*

Winter savory (mountain savory, *Satureja montana)*

ESSENTIAL OILS WITH MONOTERPENE ALCOHOLS AS MAIN ACTIVE INGREDIENT

Linalol: rosewood *(Aniba rosaeodora),* coriander *(Coriandrum sativum),* petitgrain (bitter orange leaf) *(Citrus aurantium* sp. *aurantium)*, thyme (linalol type) *(Thymus vulgaris)*

Citronellol: geranium *(Pelargonium odorantissum)*, rose *(Rose damascena)*

Geraniol: palmarosa *(Cymbopogon martini)*

α-Terpineol: *Eucalyptus radiata,* niaouli *(Melaleuca quinquenervia viridiflora,* MQV), Ravensare aromatica

Terpineol-4: tea tree *(Melaleuca alternifolia, Melaleuca linariifolia),* marjoram *(Origanum majorana)*, mastic *(Pistacia lentiscus)*

Menthol: peppermint *(Mentha piperita),* spearmint *(Mentha spicata)*

Monoterpene esters

Alcohols, including terpene alcohols, react easily with acids to form a new chemical compound: a so-called ester. In the plant world, esters are almost always strongly aromatic, often with a distinctive, fruity note.

Esters are therefore used in the flavor industry especially for foods with fruit flavors. In aromatherapy, oils with a high ester content are used for their balancing and antispasmodic effects. This antispasmodic action is dependent on the chain length of the acid half of the molecule.[12] Esters of formic acid (one carbon atom) are the main component in geranium oil, and their antispasmodic influence is only mild. Geranium *(Pelargonium)* is often used in massage oils because its gentle effect is desirable for this application.

Esters of acetic acid (two-carbon atoms), so-called acetates, can be found in everlasting, *Inula graveolens*, rosemary (verbenone type), and fir *(Abies siberica)*, as well as bay laurel and cardamom, which is a time-tested remedy for digestive cramps. Esters of acids with five carbon atoms are the main components of Roman chamomile, one of aromatherapy's strongest antispasmodics.

Esters of acids with seven carbon atoms have the strongest antispasmodic effect, and can be found in ylang ylang and in mandarin petitgrain.

Esters also act as fungicides, and are useful in preventing fungal and yeast infections. Geranium oil, which does not have a very strong antibacterial effect but is an effective fungicide, is especially significant in treating yeast infections.

ESSENTIAL OILS WITH MONOTERPENE ALDEHYDES AS MAIN ACTIVE COMPONENTS

Citronellal: eucalyptus *(Eucalyptus citriodora)*, citronella (java variety, *Cymbopogon winterianus*; ceylon variety, *Cymbopogon nardus)*

Citral: lemongrass *(Cymbopogon citratus)*, Indian verbena *(Andropogon citratus)*, lemon verbena *(Lippia citriodora)*, melissa *(Melissa officinalis)*

Monoterpene aldehydes

The citruslike aroma of melissa is well known and easy to recognize. The aldehydes responsible for this effect are citral and citronellal. They are important starting materials for the chemical industry and are extracted in large quantities from the oils of the citronella grasses.

Essential oils with a high aldehyde content have sedative and anti-inflammatory effects. The anti-inflammatory effect is most pronounced if the oil is administered in low concentrations, diluted in either air or liquid. The sedative and antispasmodic effects of citral and citronellal are stronger in relatively lower concentrations (citral is also an effective antiviral agent). Higher concentrations or doses above a certain saturation level will lessen rather than strengthen the effects. In 1973 Wagner and Sprinkmeyer[13] demonstrated this behavior of the sedative effects of various terpene compounds. Lemongrass, for example, if used undiluted, can even have a mild irritant quality.

Monoterpene ketones

The salient quality of essential oils containing ketones is the stimulating effect on cell and tissue regeneration. Applied externally, thuja oil, and especially everlasting (*Helichrysum italicum*), can give spectacular results for healing wounds or promoting the generation of new tissue. For this reason everlasting oil often is used in regenerative skin care.

An entirely different aspect of the monoterpene ketones is their mucolytic effect, in other words their ability to facilitate the loosening and elimination of mucus.

Toxicity of ketones

A variety of ketones can have toxic effects: they attack parts of the nervous system. For this reason, it is absolutely essential to use oils with a high ketone content in correct dosages (see page 44). Oils with a high thujone content, such as sage, mugwort, wormwood, thuja, and hyssop (with pinocamphone content), should be used with special caution at any time.

Because the ketone content of essential oils such as eucalyptus (*E. globulus*) or rosemary (verbenone type) is relatively unproblematic, these oils can be used for their mucolytic effects.

In general, ketones stimulate the formation of tissue, have mucolytic effects, dissolve fats, and are potentially neurotoxic.

Monoterpene oxides

A large number of essential oils contain cineole, a terpene oxide also known as eucalyptol. The characteristic structural element of this compound is an oxygen atom that is integrated into a terpene ring system. Especially high concentrations of this molecule are found in the various

ESSENTIAL OILS WITH KETONES AS MAIN COMPONENT

Pinocamphone: hyssop (*Hyssopus officinalis*)

Camphor: white camphor (*Cinnamomum camphora*)

Verbenone: rosemary, verbenone type (*Rosmarinus officinalis*)

Pinocarvone: eucalyptus (*Eucalyptus globulus*)

Piperitone: eucalyptus (*Eucalyptus dives*)

Carvone: dill (*Anethum graveolens*)

Thujone: thuja (*Thuja occidentalis*), sage (*Salvia officinalis*), wormwood (*Artemisia absinthum*)

eucalyptus and melaleuca oils. This compound has strong antiviral and expectorant (meaning it stimulates the bronchi to cough up and eliminate mucus) effects.

Interestingly, the oil of creeping hyssop (*Hyssopus officinalis* var. *decumbens*) is the only commercially available oil with a content of linalol oxide. Because of its outstanding antiviral and expectorant effects, this oil is used in aroma medicine for the treatment of bronchial infections.

Monoterpenes without functional groups: Where do they get the scent?

All citrus oils (with the exception of bergamot) contain up to 90 percent or more monoterpene hydrocarbons. The typical aroma of these oils stems not from the terpenes but from strongly aromatic trace components. Lemon oil, for example, is composed primarily of limonene. Characteristic for its aroma is the 3.5 percent content of citral. Grapefruit oil (*Citrus paradisi*) can contain up to 90 percent monoterpenes, but its characteristic aroma comes from traces of nootkatone (C15-ketone) and paramenthenthiol. Mandarin oil (*Citrus reticulata*) contains up to 90 percent monoterpenes, but its aroma comes largely from methylanthranilate, which is also responsible for mandarin's calming effects. Orange oil (*Citrus sinensis*) can contain up to 95 percent of the monoterpene limonene, but its characteristic aroma comes from sinensal (aldehyde), and a variety of other trace components.

Other important essential oils that are composed primarily of monoterpenes are pepper oil, various pine oils, nutmeg, juniper, and turpentine. Angelica oil also contains primarily monoterpenes. The warm, musky scent of angelica is brought about by macrocyclic lactones (cyclic esters) and ketones (especially pentadecanolide). These lactones and ketones make up only about 0.2 to 0.4 percent of angelica oil.

Sesquiterpenes without functional groups

The qualities of sesquiterpenes differ significantly from those of the monoterpenes. They are primarily anti-inflammatory, cooling, and antiallergenic. It is somewhat problematic to summarize the properties of these compounds in a streamlined way for the purposes of aromatherapy, because they are chemically very different. It is still reasonable, however, to characterize the effects of sesquiterpenes as anti-inflammatory and anti-allergenic. Chamazulene, which is an active component of German chamomile and has a special calming effect, and caryophyllene, which is found in various concentrations in many different oils, belong in this group.

A wide spectrum of action exists among sesquiterpenes containing functional groups with oxygen. While it was possible to classify the monoterpenes according to functional groups, this is not possible with the sesquiterpenes, because their effects are too varied to enable simple categorization. The influence of the relatively larger molecular structure equals that of the functional group.

Sesquiterpene alcohols

The interplay between chemical structure and effect is more varied with sesquiterpene alcohols than with monoterpene alcohols. The disscussion of sesquiterpene alcohols shall therefore be limited to a few well-researched examples. In general, we can characterize the effects of sesquiterpene alcohols as antiallergenic, liver stimulating, stimulating glandular secretions, and anti-inflammatory.

Bisabolol, a natural sesquiterpene alcohol, is the strongest anti-inflammatory substance in German chamomile (*Matricaria recutita*).[14] Comprehensive pharmacological studies[15] have shown that the effect of this alcohol is even stronger than that of chamazulene, which lends chamomile oil its distinctive blue color. The main components of the most valuable chemotype of German chamomile[16] are the hydrocarbons farnesene and chamazulene, as well as up to 35 percent (–)α-bisabolol, the most effective variant of this molecule.

Other plants from the Compositae family (*Asteraceae*) have proven to be a reservoir of pharmacologically active components. Echinacea (*Echinacea purpurea* and *Echinacea angustifolia*) is normally used in the form of an extract or tincture, but the essential oil derived from its roots has immune-stimulating qualities, which lately

ESSENTIAL OILS WITH SESQUITERPENE ALCOHOLS AS MAIN ACTIVE COMPONENT

(–)α-Bisabolol: German chamomile (*Matricaria recutita*)

Zingiberol: ginger (*Zingiber officinalis*)

Patchouli-alcohol: patchouli (*Pogostemon cablin*)

α-Santalol: sandalwood (*Santalum album*)

Viridiflorol: niaouli (*Melaleuca quinquenervia viridiflora*, MQV), peppermint (*Mentha piperita*), sage (*Salvia officinalis*)

have been attributed to a number of sesquiterpene alcohols.

Sandalwood is composed almost exclusively of the alcohol santalol (fifteen carbon atoms). It is traditionally used for bladder or urinary tract infections and heartburn. Authors of different studies have disagreed on its antiseptic qualities: some recommend this oil for the treatment of various urinary problems, while others have observed no therapeutic effects. One can assume that the effects of sandalwood oil are influenced more by immune-modulant properties than by antibiotic ones. Other oils with a high content of alcohols with fifteen carbon atoms are niaouli (*Melaleuca quinquenervia viridiflora*), ginger, patchouli, vetiver, carrot seed, and spikenard.

In general, sesquiterpene alcohols tonify muscles and nerves, reduce congestion in the veins as well as in the lymphatic system, and have moderate antimicrobial effects. Some of the sesquiterpene alcohols in essential oils have unique qualities: viridiflorol, found in niaouli or sage, has an estrogenlike influence and works as a tonic on the veins; spathulenol, found in verbena (*Lippia citriodora*), acts as a fungicide; cedrol, found in atlas cedar, is a tonic for the veins; santalol, found in sandalwood, is a tonic for the heart; and carotol, from carrot seed oil (*Daucus carota*), stimulates the regeneration of liver cells.

Sesquiterpene ketones and sesquiterpenes with other functional groups can have very interesting effects, but these effects vary greatly from oil to oil.

CHAPTER 3

THE EFFECTS OF ESSENTIAL OILS

Antibacterial Effects

A subject of exhaustive research at the end of the last century was the ability of essential oils to halt the spread of microorganisms. One explanation for this characteristic of essential oils is their ability to penetrate the cell membrane and influence cellular metabolism. The number of published works in this area is so high that only those relevant to aromatherapy shall be touched upon.

In 1955 Keller and Kober found essential oils effective in controlling the number of bacteria in room air.[1] They found twenty-one essential oils that, when sprayed in an enclosed area, drastically reduced or eliminated the presence of the following microorganisms: *Escherichia coli, Eberthella thyphosa, Neisseria gonorrhoeae, Streptococcus faecalis, Streptococcus pyogenes, Staphylococcus aureus, Bacillus megatherium, Corynebacterium diphtheriae,* and *Candida albicans.*

When we compare the results of the many published studies for their relevance toward actual application by humans, we encounter several problems. Many of these studies are difficult to compare as they were carried out under very different conditions. This problem was addressed not long ago by Jansen, Scheffer, and Baerheim Svendsen who compared data from forty-eight different studies published between 1976 and 1986 on the antimicrobial effects of essential oils.[2]

Of these studies, one dealt with a question of great interest in aromatherapy: the antimicrobial effect of oils of varying chemotypes of the same plant. This study compared the efficacy of various chemotypes of *Thymus vulgaris* against a variety of bacteria.

The results of this study are quite interesting. They show that in many cases thyme oils with a low phenol content, such as thyme linalol or thyme geraniol, have effects comparable to thyme oils with a higher phenol content.

The Melissengeist Study

Klosterfrau Melissengeist (spirit of melissa) is a remedy made of different essential oils according to an old traditional recipe. In an outstanding study, Wagner and Sprinkmeyer examined the pharmacological effects of the twenty main components of Klosterfrau Melissengeist.[3] Although this 1973 study does not directly address the problems and topics of aromatherapy, the results concerning the sedative, antispasmodic, and antibacterial qualities of the components examined are of great relevance because the terpenes, sesquiterpenes, and phenylpropanes examined in the study are so common in essential oils that nearly every conceivable composition of essential oils will contain a considerable

RELATIVE ANTIMICROBIAL EFFECTIVENESS OF VARIOUS CHEMOTYPES OF *THYMUS VULGARIS* OIL

	Oil					
Microorganism	Geraniol	Linalol	Terpineol	Thujanol	Carvacrol	Thymol
Staphylococcus aureus	2.5	2.5	2.5	2.5	5.0	10.0
Staphylococcus epidermitis	5.0	5.0	2.5	2.5	5.0	10.0
Micrococcus flavus	10.0	10.0	5.0	5.0	10.0	20.0
Bacillus subtilis	5.0	5.0	5.0	2.5	5.0	10.0
Escherichia coli	5.0	5.0	2.5	2.5	5.0	10.0
Klebsiella pneumoniae	5.0	5.0	2.5	2.5	5.0	10.0
Proteus vulgaris	10.0	5.0	5.0	5.0	5.0	10.0
Pseudomonas aeruginosa	0.625	0.625	0.625	0.625	0.625	1.25
Candida albicans	20.0	5.0	5.0	5.0	5.0	10.0

0 = ineffective, 20 = highly effective

MAIN COMPONENTS OF KLOSTERFRAU MELISSENGEIST

Components	Found in
Caryophyllene	clove
Citral	melissa, lemongrass, may chang (*Litsea cubeba*)
Eugenol	clove, laurel
Eugenol acetate	clove
Limonene	all citrus oils
Linalol	lavender, neroli, coriander
Terpineol	niaouli, cajeput, eucalyptus varieties
Cinnamic aldehyde	cinnamon bark
Citronellol	geranium, rose
Citronellal	citronella, *Eucalyptus citriodora*
Geraniol	palmarosa
Linalyl acetate	lavender, clary sage

this group of illnesses (Group 2).

The results are quite surprising. In the words of the authors:

> The results of our research showed that, with varying degrees of intensity, there was an inhibiting influence on all the bacteria tested, especially those primarily associated with bronchopneumonial conditions. The large spectrum of this inhibitory action is as broad as, or even greater than, that of wide-spectrum antibiotics.

The Aromatogram

Paul Belaiche, in his three-volume work *Traité de Phytothérapie et d'Aromathérapie* (Treatise on

amount of at least some of them.

The authors discovered that the essential oils that make up Klosterfrau Melissengeist are to varying degrees effective against all the microorganisms listed in the box to the right.

Of special interest were the results relevant to microorganisms associated with bronchitis or bronchopneumonial conditions. The authors distinguish between the main microorganisms associated with these conditions (Group 1) and microorganisms less frequently associated with

EFFECTIVENESS OF MELISSENGEIST TERPENES AGAINST VARIOUS AGENTS THAT CAUSE ILLNESSES OF THE LUNGS AND BRONCHIAL SYSTEM

Group I, primary:

Pneumococcus spec., *Klebsiella pneumoniae, Staphylococcus aureus haemolyticus, Neisseria catarrhalis, Streptococcus haemolyticus, Proteus vulgaris, Haemophilus influenzae, Haemophilus pertussis*

Group 2, secondary:

Candida albicans, Escherichia coli—Aerobacter group, various *Corynebacteria, Listeria*

Phytotherapy and Aromatherapy), made a decisive advance for the practical application of the antimicrobial qualities of essential oils.[4] Belaiche describes the basic aspects of using essential oils to treat infectious illnesses. In thousands of tests and countless clinical cases, he investigated the effectiveness of essential oils in treating a wide range of conditions.

Belaiche used the aromatogram, a testing method that allowed him to examine the effectiveness of essential oils against specific bacteria. These microbiological tests are used in aromamedicine (a term that refers to the medicinal uses of aromatherapy) to determine the most effective essential oil combination for combating a specific infection. Cultures of a patient's intestinal flora are exposed to various essential oils to determine which essential oils have the strongest antibacterial effects against the pathogens specific to a particular patient. From the information derived from thousands of aromatograms some generalizations can be made regarding the effectiveness of essential oils against various pathogenic bacteria. In his book, Belaiche examines the sensitivity of pathogenic germs to a variety of essential oils. His work contains comprehensive tables that list the degree of effectiveness of forty essential oils against the pathogens occurring most frequently in common infectious diseases: *Proteus morgani*, *Proteus mirabilis*, *Proteus rettgeri* (intestinal infection), *Alcalescens dispar*, *Corynebacterium xerosa* (diphtheria), *Neisseria flava* (sinus and ear infection), *Klebsiella pneumoniae* (lung infection), *Staphylococcus alba* (food poisoning), *Staphylococcus aureus* (pus-causing), and *Pneumococcus*, *Candida albicans*.

The aromatogram gives us a graphic depiction of the effectiveness of essential oils: the bacteria-free area around the drops of oregano oil shows its effectiveness against a specific bacterium.

Ginger

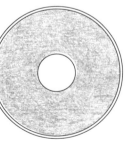

Geranium

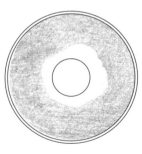

Oregano

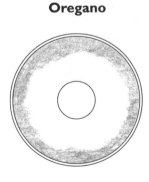

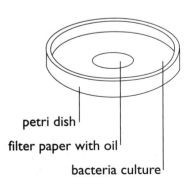

petri dish

filter paper with oil

bacteria culture

Bacteria spread without inhibition.

Bacteria spread except to the small area surrounding the filter paper.

Bacteria can survive only on the edge of the petri dish.

EFFECTIVENESS OF ESSENTIAL OILS AGAINST MICROORGANISMS

Numerical values indicate the measure of sensivitivity of each microorganism to the oils (0 = no reaction; 1 = inhibition).

Essential oil	Proteus	Enterococcus	Staphylococcus	Streptococcus	Pneumococcus	Alcalescens dispar	Neisseria	Corynebacterium xerosa	Klebsiella	Candida	Aromatic Index
Atlas cedar	0.07	0.13	0.00	0.00	0.00	0.00	0.00	0.09	0.00	0.00	0.03
Basil	0.00	0.00	0.02	0.00	0.04	0.00	0.00	0.07	0.00	0.00	0.01
Bergamot	0.00	0.00	0.02	0.00	0.00	0.00	0.05	0.07	0.14	0.00	0.03
Bergamot, neroli	0.18	0.21	0.01	0.11	0.00	0.16	0.01	0.09	0.14	0.09	0.09
Bergamot, petitgrain	0.09	0.23	0.16	0.22	0.20	0.16	0.15	0.04	0.25	0.77	0.17
Cajeput	0.33	0.30	0.33	0.11	0.50	0.04	0.15	0.04	0.00	0.00	0.02
Chamomile, Roman	0.00	0.00	0.01	0.00	0.00	0.00	0.00	0.00	0.00	0.00	0.00
Cinnamon	0.73	0.65	0.86	0.77	0.67	0.30	0.90	0.69	0.78	0.67	0.69
Citronella	0.06	0.06	0.01	0.00	0.00	0.13	0.00	0.11	0.05	0.00	0.04
Clove	0.33	0.52	0.60	0.44	0.83	0.73	0.59	0.38	0.33	0.40	0.52
Coriander	0.00	0.00	0.02	0.00	0.08	0.00	0.00	0.03	0.19	0.00	0.05
Cypress	0.00	0.03	0.00	0.16	0.00	0.00	0.00	0.04	0.00	0.03	0.03
Eucalyptus	0.35	0.16	0.39	0.00	0.45	0.33	0.27	0.40	0.39	0.30	0.31
Geranium	0.12	0.20	0.33	0.28	0.38	0.13	0.31	0.09	0.05	0.02	0.19
Hyssop	0.00	0.04	0.00	0.11	0.00	0.00	0.00	0.00	0.00	0.00	0.01
Juniper	0.03	0.01	0.02	0.00	0.00	0.00	0.00	0.04	0.00	0.05	0.02
Laurel	0.04	0.00	0.02	0.16	0.00	0.00	0.09	0.11	0.11	0.00	0.03
Lavender	0.20	0.36	0.25	0.61	0.33	0.13	0.19	0.23	0.30	0.26	0.03
Lemon	0.06	0.12	0.09	0.00	0.12	0.13	0.13	0.07	0.00	0.05	0.09
Lemongrass	0.00	0.00	0.04	0.00	0.08	0.00	0.00	0.00	0.11	0.00	0.02
Myrtle	0.27	0.16	0.27	0.00	0.33	0.46	0.25	0.50	0.39	0.13	0.25
Niaouli	0.21	0.21	0.03	0.16	0.00	0.16	0.00	0.00	0.08	0.05	0.10
Nutmeg	0.00	0.00	0.00	0.00	0.04	0.00	0.00	0.11	0.11	0.00	0.03
Oregano	0.92	0.78	0.92	0.83	0.96	0.10	0.92	0.88	0.78	0.78	0.87
Peppermint	0.02	0.09	0.01	0.11	0.12	0.06	0.00	0.07	0.03	0.12	0.07
Pine	0.29	0.33	0.40	0.28	0.41	0.40	0.21	0.40	0.30	0.26	0.32
Rosemary	0.12	0.04	0.12	0.16	0.12	0.00	0.00	0.00	0.03	0.11	0.08
Sage	0.00	0.00	0.00	0.16	0.08	0.16	0.00	0.00	0.00	0.02	0.04
Savory	0.24	0.28	0.72	0.50	0.50	0.40	0.60	0.71	0.39	0.33	0.46
Spike lavender	0.23	0.19	0.09	0.00	0.04	0.06	0.00	0.20	0.08	0.03	0.09
Tarragon	0.06	0.12	0.22	0.16	0.20	0.00	0.09	0.16	0.25	0.13	0.14
Thyme	0.74	0.72	0.65	0.66	0.92	1.00	0.64	0.64	0.42	0.70	0.71
Verbena	0.00	0.00	0.08	0.00	0.00	0.00	0.005	0.04	0.00	0.00	0.02

The effectiveness of essential oils against these germs was observed not only in laboratory tests. Belaiche also clinically treated numerous infectious illnesses, among them chronic and acute bronchitis, rhinitis (cold, catarrh), angina, sinus infection, bladder infection, intestinal infections, skin infections, childhood illnesses, tuberculosis, and malaria.

In a summary of his results, Belaiche divides the forty essential oils into three groups according to microbicidal strength: The first group, with the broadest spectrum of efficacy, consists of oregano, savory, cinnamon, thyme, and clove (Belaiche later added tea tree oil to this group).

The second group consists of oils that are effective only against certain classes of bacteria. In this group we find pine oil, cajeput, *Eucalyptus globulus*, lavender, myrtle, geranium, petitgrain, tarragon, niaouli, and *Thymus serpyllium*.

Belaiche defined a third group of oils in which a direct influence on bacteria was observed seldom or only irregularly. Belaiche attributed the healing effects that are nonetheless observed in these oils to effects on the bodily terrain. He concluded that these oils affect the immune response, which in turn makes it impossible for the bacteria to spread.

The Special Role of Tea Tree Oil

Belaiche published his results at a time when tea tree (*Melaleuca alternifolia, M. linarifolia*) oil was still not widely known. In later studies, Belaiche supplemented his findings on the antibacterial effects of essential oils with extensive work on the clinical efficacy of tea tree oil. He focused on tea tree oil's effectiveness in treating infections of the skin and urogenital tract. He tested the effectiveness of tea tree oil for the treatment of bladder infection as follows: Patients were given 8 milligrams of tea tree oil in stomach acid–resistant gelatin capsules three times daily. Symptoms related to bladder infection disappeared in 60 percent of the Patients. Liver function was also monitored during the six-month treatment period and did not show deviation from normal levels, as is usually the case during treatment with antibiotics.

Another series of tests dealt with patients having vaginitis caused by *Candida albicans*. Patients were treated with vaginal gelatin capsules. The dosage was 0.2 gram of tea tree oil in a 2-gram gelatin capsule. Capsules were administered before bedtime for ninety days. Out of 27 patients, 23 recovered fully; symptoms of vaginal discharge and burning sensations stopped entirely. Microbiological tests showed the disappearance of *Candida albicans* in 21 of 27 patients.

Belaiche attributed these noteworthy results to two factors:

1. the strong antimicrobial effect of tea tree oil itself, which is evident in the aromatogram, and
2. tea tree oil's extreme tolerability, which allows its use for long periods of time without the slightest irritation to mucous membranes.

Belaiche's work continued Gattefossé's allopathic tradition: the pathogenic microorganism is opposed by active components of essential oils, identified as the phenols and cinnamic aldehydes in thyme, oregano, savory, clove, and cinnamon.

There are many successful treatments with the above-named oils, but also disappointing results where the highly esteemed "broad spectrum antibiotics" of aromatherapy proved inexplicably ineffective. Surprisingly it is often possible with these highly active oils to treat a disease symptomatically, as is done in conventional medicine. If this does not succeed, and the symptoms cannot be effectively countered, then the holistic approach may be more effective. What is needed is not merely the removal of symptoms, but addressing the cause, that is, healing the whole person.

Combining Scientific and Holistic Approaches

A physician who is an exemplary advocate and practitioner of this view is Daniel Pénoël. Originally known for his collaboration with Pierre Franchomme and their work *L'Aromathérapie exactement*, Pénoël is today one of the leading proponents of an aromamedicine that derives its superiority through the combination of proper use of scientific results with holistic, patient-oriented healing. With regard to the treatment of infectious illnesses, Pénoël summarizes the special conditions of the scientific-holistic approach as follows:[5]

> Every individual has his or her own unique set of bacteria, even if they may not seem morphologically different from that of the next person. A streptococcus from person A, however, is not necessarily identical to a streptococcus of the same type in person B.
>
> The more serious and chronic a case, the more exceptional and unexpected are the essential oils that turn out to be effective.

If an active oil is found, then its properties may point to possible hidden causes of the illness.

The effects of essential oils are in every case multifaceted and deep, and principally different from the one-dimensional effects of antibiotics. . . .

Where antibiotics inflict extensive damage on human bacterial flora, essential oils respect the integrity of necessary "friendly" bacteria of the organism, a condition for true and lasting healing.

Clearly the healing powers of essential oils can be put to be0st use when the body of knowledge of the pharmacology of oils is combined with a modern, holistic sensitivity. A case from the practice of Dr. Pénoël illustrates this:

> In the case of a patient with a lengthy upper respiratory tract infection, oils such as oregano were not effective against those bacteria against which they are usually successfully employed. Following observations that the patient also suffered from varicose veins, mastic oil (*Pistacia lentiscus*) was tested in an aromatogram and unexpectedly proved effective against the pathogenic germs. This example illustrates vividly how ordinary principles do not always lead to the best treatment, and that substances that may be totally ineffective for many may provide the best treatment for a specific patient.

Antiviral Effects

It has been known for quite some time that certain plant extracts exert a more or less powerful

ANTIVIRAL OILS AND THEIR COMPONENTS

Component	Oils[a]
β-Caryophyllene	found in many oils, such as lavender, rosemary, and thyme (linalol type)
Limonene	all citrus oils
α-Sabines	in many oils, such as tea tree and laurel
γ-Terpinene	in many oils, especially juniper, eucalyptus, niaouli, and tea tree, among others
Eugenol	clove (Ocimum gratissimum[b])
Cinnamic aldehyde	cinnamon bark
Anethol	anise
Linalol	in many oils, such as lavender and neroli
Linalyl acetate	in many oils, such as clary sage, lavender, and bergamot
Carvone	dill
Citral	in many oils, such as melissa, Litsea cubeba, and lemongrass
Citronellol	rose, geranium

a. Black pepper, cassia, and cardamom were also proven effective.

b. Ocimum gratissimum is related to basil but, like clove oil, has a higher concentration of eugenol.

antiviral effect. In studying extracts of over one hundred plants from the Lamiaceae family, the great majority were found to have antiviral effects.[6]

These results led to the development of a cream used in the treatment of herpes (this preparation is sold in Germany under the name Lomaherpan), the active ingredient of which is an extract of melissa. At the time of this development, the aromatherapy books by Dr. Jean Valnet and Robert Tisserand had already become classics in Germany. These authors recommend bergamot, eucalyptus, geranium, and lemon. Other authors have recommended additional oils for the treatment of herpes:

- Pénoël: niaouli, eucalyptus
- Franchomme: tea tree
- Belaiche: cypress
- Wagner: rose, melissa

Impressive scientific studies have confirmed the antiviral effects of essential oils. A study of fundamental importance for aromatherapy by

R. Deiniger and A. Lembke, presented in 1987 at the first International Congress for Phytotherapy in Cologne, demonstrated the effectiveness of three oils and approximately fifteen common oil components against herpes and adenovirus (organisms that cause diseases of the respiratory tract and gastroenteritis with a respiratory tract infection).[7]

It can be concluded that each of the classes of essential oil components present in essential oils, terpene hydrocarbons, and terpenes with functional groups such as aldehydes, ketones, or alcohols and also phenylpropane derivatives show effectiveness against viruses.

The choice of compounds made by Deiniger and Lembke for this study reflects the experience of the scientists; with respect to aromatherapy, however, the choice of compounds is arbitrary. For example, if citronellol has an antiviral effect, there is no reason why geraniol should not be as effective.

This conclusion is also reflected in the treatments recommended by aromatherapy authors. That essential oils generally display varying degrees of effectiveness against viruses is supported by more studies that describe the effectiveness of oils against influenza, mumps, chicken pox, and polio viruses and by experiences gathered in aromatherapy in which the effectiveness of essential oils against herpes and shingles is unsurpassed.

As shown by Indians of the Pacific Northwest, placing more faith in a much broader effectiveness of essential oils against viral illnesses is more justified than the paucity of scientific studies would suggest. These Indians were able to protect themselves against the devastating consequences of the worldwide flu epidemic of 1918 with a preparation made from a native plant, *Lomatium dissectum*.[8] Today this plant is experiencing a renaissance in alternative medicine in the U.S. because of its antiviral effects.

Another example illustrates how modern science and today's society in general can learn from Native people: interestingly enough, it was also the North American Indians from whom Western medicine learned to use echinacea (*Echinacea purpurea*) as an immune booster, and today Echinacea tinctures are a staple of many household medicine cabinets.

Knowledge of the wide spectrum of action of essential oils against viruses runs hand in hand with observations noting that the behavior of these oils is not necessarily just a result of their unique chemical compositions, but potentially stems from their remarkable ability to penetrate cell membranes and their lipophilic character.[9]

Inhalation and Expectorant Effects

In an earlier study, E. M. Boyd and his coworkers tested the expectorant properties of a large number of essential oils.[10] As a measure of expectoration the quantity and consistency of bronchial fluids were determined.

Boyd measured the changes in specific weight, the percentage of solid components, and especially the content of soluble mucus. Boyd defined the term *bronchial fluid*, which includes secretions of the alveoli (the air sacs, or air-containing cells, of the lungs), the trachea, and the bronchial tubes. Increased secretion and an increased concentration of mucus in the secretion were termed *expectorant effect*.

Boyd found that, when inhaled, the following oils have expectorant effects: nutmeg, thuja, lemon, anise, citronella, palmarosa, pine, fennel, thyme, and eucalyptus. Essential oils are most effectively used for a dry, nervous cough.

In addition, Boyd distinguished between systemic and local expectorants and determined that oils taken orally produced no discernible effects. Inhalation of oils, on the other hand, even in very small doses, led to positive results.

It was observed further that the desired effects were drastically minimized, or even negated, when the dosage applied was so high that the air inhaled had a noticeable aroma. For inhalation, only minimal doses should be used, just enough to produce a very faint scent. Increasing concentrations change a secretion-stimulating effect into a secretion-inhibiting effect.

Another clinical study determined the terpene levels in the blood of test subjects after they inhaled essential oils. It was found that through inhalation, the components of essential oils reached therapeutically active levels.[11]

Within thirty to forty minutes the concentration of essential oils absorbed through inhalation sinks to half its original value. This demonstrates that there is no danger of accumulating essential oils in the body even with repeated use.

Sedative and Antispasmodic Effects

Essential oils have been used traditionally for their sedative and antispasmodic effects, thoroughly described throughout aromatherapy literature. Scientific data from animal tests appear interesting but are unsatisfying. On the one hand, they have confirmed many of aromatherapy's most deeply held concepts; on the other hand, a direct translation to human use is problematic.

Interestingly, clinical results in clear support of essential oils, though rare, were in fact established already in the 1970s. At that time it was possible to convincingly demonstrate the effectiveness of, again, the main components of Klosterfrau Melissengeist for imbalances of the autonomic nervous system in a double-blind study.[12] Over 80 percent of the patients reported good to very good results in the therapy of nervousness, anxiety, depression, inner tension, headaches, dizziness, heaviness in the legs, general exhaustion, fatigue, insomnia, and loss of appetite.[13,14]

Sedative Effects

These results have been supported by further studies on the individual components of essential oils. The sesquiterpene caryophyllene proved to be the most effective of all the substances tested.[15] Investigating the main components of melissa oil, the alcohols citronellol and geraniol, as well as the aldehydes citronellal and citral showed that citronellal had the strongest sedative effects. Citral was nearly as effective, while geraniol and citronellol were, as expected, practically without effect. The study found that nearly all of the terpenes and phenylpropane derivatives tested possessed very good sedative qualities when administered orally.

The study also concluded that no direct correlation between the type of chemical compound (such as alcohols, ketones, etc.) and efficacy of

COMPOUNDS TESTED AND SHOWN TO HAVE SIGNIFICANT SEDATIVE EFFECTS

Caryophyllene, citral, citronellal, estragol, eugenol, eugenyl acetate, linalol, linalyl acetate, linalyl butyrate, linalyl isovalerate, methyl eugenol, clove oil

the substances tested can be observed.

Most of the oil components tested had their strongest effects with the lowest of the tested doses, which was 1 milligram per kilogram of body weight. For a body weight of 70 kilograms this would correspond to a dosage of 70 milligrams, or two to five drops. For the most part, raising the dosage resulted in a reduction of effectiveness, which is also confirmed by experiences in aromatherapy.

If, twenty years after these studies, one were to correlate the components and the oils in which they are predominately found, it would become obvious that experiences in practical aromatherapy are in accordance with the scientific data. The citronellal of melissa and *Eucalyptus citriodora* and the linalol found in lavender are among the components with the strongest sedative effects.

Also, limonene of lemon has a significant calming effect. Oils derived from melissa, *Eucalyptus citriodora*, lemon verbena, citronella, and other oils with a high aldehyde content also have a strong sedative effect.[16]

Antispasmodic Effects

Tarragon and basil oil are distinguished by their special effects on the autonomic nervous system and the digestive tract. The phenylpropane ethers, especially estragole (methyl chavicol), stabilize an overactive sympathetic nervous system (sympatholytic effect) and restore a healthy balance between the sympathetic and the parasympathetic nervous systems. The antispasmodic effect of these oils is—as evidenced by their culinary usage—especially pronounced in the digestive organs. The traditional use of Pernod, Ouzo, and other anise-flavored liqueurs after a heavy meal is a familiar example of these effects.

As for their effects on the central nervous system and stress-related symptoms, oils with a high ester content, such as clary sage and Roman chamomile, are equally effective antispasmodics. They reduce tension in stressful situations or with premenstrual discomfort.

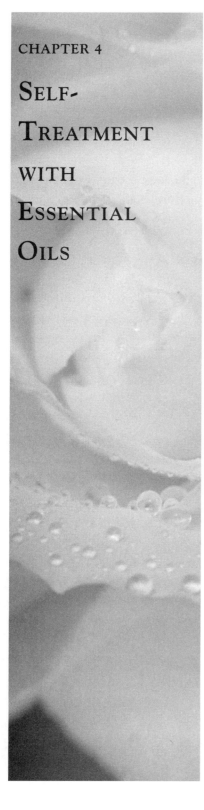

CHAPTER 4

SELF-TREATMENT WITH ESSENTIAL OILS

A word of caution: In no case should enthusiasm for aromatherapy, or any form of self-treatment, preclude seeing a doctor or other qualified health-care provider if the condition requires.

Real and Potential Risks

Before discussing the particulars of the properties and uses of essential oils in detail, it is wise to address some common questions that arise over and over with regard to their use in self-medication. To begin with, a statement from the man who certainly did more for the growing popularity of aromatherapy than anyone else, Dr. Jean Valnet:

> No, in contrast to what many doctors say—some of my students among them—who only think of protecting their monopoly and filling their pockets, I do not believe that it is necessary to be a doctor to use aromatherapy. Naturally, it is necessary to know the intensity of essential oils to avoid errors. Thousands of individuals treat themselves

without adverse side effects by following the proper dosages I have outlined.

It is a given that every human activity presents certain risks. If essential oils are used arbitrarily and applied in excess, it is possible that some may burn or sting or cause allergic reactions, and some might actually be harmful. If, however, we use essential oils responsibly and with common sense, the risks are minimal. Proper dosage is as critical for plant-derived medications and essential oils as for any other drugs. Any form of medication, whether a conventional drug or essential oil, that has positive effects when administered in a therapeutic dosage can cause severe problems if overdosed.

Nevertheless, the risks associated with plant medicines have been exaggerated by the pharmaceutical lobby, as statistics show. According to the American Association of Poison Control Centers, 809 cases of fatal poisonings and 6,407 cases of serious but nonfatal poisonings were reported caused by conventional pharmaceuticals between 1988 and 1989. In contrast, plant-based preparations caused 2 fatalities and 53 serious poisonings in the same time period. The most dangerous plants were not medicinal but were house plants or shrubs.[1]

Toxicity of Essential Oils

While the appropriate use of essential oils is normally free of any complications, there are some toxic effects of essential oils that have to be recognized and avoided. If used in an appropriate, sensible manner, essential oils are safe and their use should be free of any complications.

As opposed to conventional medicine, which promises quick results and, especially, safe medications, we are left to our own devices or to the consultation of published studies to assess the potential toxicity of essential oils. There are very few accessible studies on the toxicity of essential oils, and only one standard work that compiles available data for the purposes of aromatherapy: Robert Tisserand's *The Essential Oil Safety Data Manual.*

Evaluating toxicological data, even the majority of those found in the *Safety Data Manual,* can only provide certain clues that are based on studies evaluating the potential risks of using those oils within the context of cosmetic products. Much of these data from the cosmetics industry are so-called LD-50 values for mice, which means the dose of a given substance that proves fatal for 50 percent of the test animals. These results are only of limited value when applied to human use.

Essential oils containing ketones: Neurotoxic

Ketones are the most common toxic substances in essential oils. According to Pénoël, ketone molecules can penetrate the blood-brain barrier more easily than other molecules.[2] The neurotoxic epilepsy-causing effects of essential oils with a high ketone content have been documented. These oils can also cause irreversible liver damage. Therefore, these oils can only be used with appropriate caution. Total avoidance of these oils is by no means necessary, especially in view of their many desirable effects, because they can be used safely. Moreover, not all ketones encountered in essential oils are toxic, such as the fenchone of fennel oil.

Thujone is the most widely distributed ketone found in essential oils. It is found in, among others, mugwort, sage, thuja, wormwood, and yarrow oil. Mugwort and thuja contain particularly high levels of thujone and should be used with appropriate caution. The safest of all oils having a high thujone content, sage is the most common. Its frequent use points to a relatively low toxicity and there is evidence that sage oil is less toxic than the thujone it contains, were the thujone taken as an isolated substance. Experience suggests that, as with any oils containing ketones, sage oil should not be used by children or pregnant or nursing women.

Aside from some exotic oils, essential oils containing ketones are the ones with the greatest potential risk. But since we do not want to forgo these oils because of their mucolytic and cosmetic properties, the ability to use them safely should be a part of every aromatherapy user's know-how.

According to Pénoël and Franchomme, ketone toxicity depends foremost on how it is administered. The means of delivery in order of decreasing toxicity are: oral, rectal, vaginal, percutaneous, inhalation.

According to Pénoël and Franchomme, the dosages that follow on page 46 can be considered safe for oral application (values given are for the amount of essential oil, not for pure ketone).

OILS CONTAINING KETONES

Very high ketone content: All of these oils have neurotoxic and abortive effects.

Oil	Ketone	Comments
Rue (*Ruta graveolens*)	Methyl nonyl ketone	*Poisonous!* Normally not used.
Santolina (*Santolina chamaecyparisius*)	Artemisia ketone	Use is *not advisable.*
Mugwort (*Artemisia herba alba*)	Thujone	*Poisonous!* High thujone content.
Thuja (*Thuja occidentalis*)	Thujone	Nonproblematic in *small* doses administered externally.
Wormwood (*Artemisia absinthum*)	Thujone	Used to manufacture absinthe.
Hyssop (*Hyssopus officinalis*)	Pinocamphone	Use externally only with the utmost caution.
Pennyroyal (*Mentha pulegium*)	Pulegone	*Poisonous* in large doses. Avoid overdose.
Crested lavender (*Lavandula stoechas*)	Camphor	Can be confused for lavender. *Absolutely unsuitable for children.*

OILS CONTAINING KETONES (continued)

Moderate ketone content: These oils should be used with caution.

Oil	Ketone	Comments
Sage (*Salvia officinalis*)	Thujone	Appears less toxic than its thujone content would indicate. *Dangerous for children.*
Spike lavender (*Lavandula latifolia*)	Camphor	Best when mixed with benign oils.
Camphor (*Cinnamomum camphora*)	Camphor	Neurotoxic. Induces abortion.

Low ketone content: Minimal danger of toxicity when used with caution.

Oil	Ketone	Comments
Yarrow (*Achillea millefolium*)	Thujone	Caution with children.
Rosemary (camphor chemotype) (*Rosmarinus officinalis*)	Camphor	Nontoxic in small doses.
Peppermint (*Mentha piperita*)	Methone	Nontoxic in small doses. Caution with small children.
Eucalyptus polybractea (cryptone chemotype) *Eucalyptus dives* (piperitone chemotype)	Cryptone	Nontoxic if mixed with other oils.
Atlas cedar (*Cedrus atlantica*)	Atlantone	External use. Nontoxic.

Relatively problem-free oils with ketone content.

Oil	Ketone	Comments
Everlasting (*Helichrysum italicum*)	Italidione	Suitable for external use. Use internally only in very small doses.
Rosemary (verbenone chemotype) (*Rosmarinus officinalis*)	Verbenone	Suitable for external use. Use internally only in very small doses.
Eucalyptus (*Eucalyptus globulus*)	Pinocarvone	Benign.
Vetiver (*Vetiveria zizanoides*)	Vetivone	Nontoxic.

Maximum three times daily:

Adults	75 mg (approx. 3 drops)
Older children	50 mg (approx. 2 drops)
Small children	25 mg (approx. 1 drop)

The authors recommend the following dosages for percutaneous applications.

Maximum five times daily:

Adults	0.5 ml (approx. 15 drops)
Older children	0.25 ml (approx. 7 drops)
Small children	0.1 ml (approx. 3 drops)

The table on pages 44 and 45 gives an overview of the most important ketone-containing oils in aro-matherapy and a qualitative estimate of potential risks.

Oils containing phenol: Liver toxicity

Oils containing phenols are occasionally taken internally for their strong antibacterial properties. This is not problematic if doses are kept low. At high dosages, these oils may be damaging to the liver. But also in low dosages if used internally over long periods of time, these oils can cause changes in liver enzyme counts. Therefore, when necessary, these oils should be used only in the form of a short, high-intensity therapy—two to four days—which is usually well tolerated.

Harmful effects to the kidneys

One of the most well-known toxic effects is juniper oil's irritation of the kidney. Since the stimulating effect is linked to kidney-tissue damage, therapeutic use of juniper oil should be undertaken with the utmost caution. The compounds responsible for irritating the kidneys are monoterpenes. A directive published by the former German Health Ministry therefore demands that juniper oil should be made out of only the plant's berries, as such an oil contains virtually no monoterpenes, and the terpene alcohols they contain instead are nonirritant.

The discussion of kidney irritation in the study mentioned has been limited to juniper oil, but the question remains whether all oils with high levels of terpene hydrocarbons need to be more closely examined for their effects on the kidneys. Oils with 80 or 90 percent terpene hydrocarbon content are the most lipophilic of all oils. More hydrophilic molecules, like monoterpene alcohols, put less of a strain on the kidneys.

Because the kidneys have a better tolerance for oils with a high terpene alcohol or ester content—such as lavender, clary sage, or tea tree—these oils are preferred for frequent use in basic hygiene and showering.

Carcinogenic effects

After calamus and sassafras oils were fed to rats for a period of twelve months carcinogenic effects were observed. These experiments should be viewed as curiosities, and one need not panic at the sight of a bottle of sassafras oil. Validity of these experiments with respect to normal human use is limited because they rely on massive overdoses.

Recently, it has been proposed that estragole and therefore also basil oil (which contains considerable quantities of estragole) can be carcinogenic. Should these concerns be true they would also have to apply to tarragon oil, which has an estragole content of 80 percent. It has been shown that administering 500 milligrams of

PHENOL-CONTAINING OILS

Oil	Ketone	Comments
Savory (*Satureja* spec.)	Carvacrol/Thymol	Internal use in doses of less than 0.1 milliliter (approx. 3 drops) acceptable. Not for external use.
Oregano (*Oreganum vulgaris, O. compactum*)	Carvacrol	Internal use in doses of less than 0.1 milliliter (approx. 3 drops) acceptable. Best when not used externally, but if necessary, use only on the soles of the feet.
Thyme (*Thymus vulgaris*)	Carvacrol/Thymol	Internal use in doses of less than 0.1 milliliter (approx. 3 drops) nontoxic. Best when not used externally, but if necessary, use only on the soles of the feet.
Clove leaf oil (*Syzygium aromaticum*)	Eugenol	Can lead to dangerous skin irritation.

estragole per 2 pounds of body weight can cause liver cancer in rats and mice. In this case not estragole itself is the carcinogen but a metabolite formed in the body. The formation of this metabolite depends on the dosage of estragole. This leaves the possibility that the metabolite is not produced at all if estragole is introduced in minor amounts.

If these proportions were applied directly to humans, it would mean that (assuming a body weight of, say, 140 pounds) a dosage of 30 grams of estragole per day, or approximately 40 grams of basil or tarragon oil, would be required to reproduce these conditions. Again, these studies subjected animals to extremely high dosages of single substances over extremely long periods of time, dosages that far exceed the recommended dosages for humans.

Essential Oils and the Skin

Clove oil, clove leaf oil, cinnamon bark oil, and cinnamon leaf oil are currently being hotly discussed in England. These and other oils have the potential, especially with individuals predisposed toward developing allergic reactions to certain oils, to cause unpleasant or even painful skin reactions, or even to lead to dangerous and difficult-to-control complications such as swelling over the entire body and severe shortness of breath. Testing for individual tolerance of these oils before use is therefore essential (see next page).

Two types of skin reactions are possible:

1. Non-Immunological Reactions: Irritation
Non-immunological reactions are caused by so-called irritants, such as stinging nettle. They cause itching or, in higher doses, even burning. The

SIGNIFICANT SKIN-IRRITATING OILS

Oil	Irritant	Comments
Clove leaf	Eugenol	Can cause serious complications.
Clove flower	Eugenol	Less aggressive than clove leaf, but irritating nonetheless.
Cinnamon	Cinnamic aldehyde	Can cause major irritation.
Cinnamon leaves	Cinnamic aldehyde	More aggressive than cinnamon.
Cassia	Carvacrol	Can cause major irritation.
Oregano	Carvacrol/Thymol	Not for external use; internal use only in small doses.
Thyme	Carvacrol/Thymol	Not as aggressive as oregano; avoid external use.
Savory	Carvacrol/Thymol	Not for external use; internal use only in small doses.

reaction to these substances is dose-dependent: the more contact the skin has with the substance, the more severe the irritation. A number of oils, especially those with a high phenol content— such as oregano, thyme, or savory—cause such irritation if used inappropriately.

2. Immunological Reactions: Allergies
Immunological skin reactions develop based on individual tolerance for the substances in one's environment. If one has hypersensitivity to a particular substance the body responds upon first contact by producing antibodies; it becomes sensitized. With each subsequent contact, the body recognizes the substance immediately and responds with a specific skin reaction. Among essential oils, cinnamon and clove can provoke a serious allergic reaction (rashes, swelling, blistering) in susceptible individuals even in small quantities. These oils also can provoke irritation in nonallergic individuals. As little as 2 percent cinnamic aldehyde in Vaseline can provoke irritation.

Potential Sensitization to Essential Oil Components

Compared with other substances of the plant world, cinnamic aldehyde only ranks as a medium-strength contact-allergen; however, in the realm of aromatherapy it is the strongest sensitizing agent. Likewise, eugenol has considerable sensitization potential. Sensitized individuals who use cinnamon or cassia oils (cinnamic aldehyde), clove oil (eugenol), or other oils with similar compositions run the risk of developing contact dermatitis, often with serious complications, such as inflammation of the skin, possibly over the entire body, and shortness of breath. It is therefore necessary that individuals test for potential sensitivity to a specific oil by placing a small amount of the oil on the inside of the elbow and waiting 24 hours to be sure that no allergic reaction has appeared. It is advisable to test again after 24 to 48 hours to detect beginning sensitization.

To entirely take these oils out of circulation or to advise a user to avoid them completely is

PHOTOSENSITIZING OILS

Botanical family	Oils	Strength of effects
Apiaceae	*Ammi visnaga*	■ ■
	Angelica	■ ■
	Celery	■
	Parsley	■
	Tarragon	■
	Tagetes	■ ■
Lamiaceae	Lavender	■
Rutaceae	Lemon	■
	Orange	■
	Mandarin	■
	Bergamot	■

(■ = significant, ■ ■ = strong effect)

KNOWN CONTRAINDICATIONS

Condition	Do not use
Abdominal pain	clove
Asthma	yarrow, marjoram, oregano, rosemary
Breast cancer	cypress, angelica, sage, fennel, anise, caraway
Epilepsy	hyssop, sage, fennel, parsley, nutmeg, anise
Glaucoma	thyme, hyssop, cypress, tarragon
Hemorrhaging	lavender in combination with an anticoagulant
High blood pressure	lemon, hyssop
Hypothyroidism	fennel
Insomnia	peppermint, pine
Menstrual complaints	cypress, sage, angelica, anise, caraway
Prostate cancer	*Thymus serpyllum*, cypress, angelica, hyssop
Tumors	fennel, anise, caraway
Urinary tract infection	juniper, eucalyptus

equivalent to throwing the baby out with the bathwater. Clove oil, for instance, offers more than only those properties that require extreme caution. There are studies that demonstrate the anti-inflammatory qualities of clove oil. It is so effective that drops can represent a massive over-dose—potentially causing a severe skin reaction. I have found that clove oil diluted in alcohol at a 1:1,000 to 1:10,000 ratio will best provide the oil's positive effects without provoking skin irritation.

Another class of substances with relatively high sensitizing potential, sesquiterpene-lactones are found in less common oils such as costusroot or massoi, but also in yarrow, *Inula graveolens*, and laurel oil. Sensitization is also possible with common components such as geraniol, linalyl acetate, or citral; however, it is extremely rare. Similarly allergic reactions reported for Roman and German chamomile oils are caused almost exclusively by impurities in the oils or other factors and not by components of the oils themselves.[3]

Reports from older studies on the allergenic effects of oils with high levels of terpene hydrocarbons show that it is not the terpenes themselves but terpene hydroperoxides that are to blame for these reactions. Strongly irritating citrus or needle oils should therefore no longer be used if they cause a skin reaction.

Photosensitivity

Essential oils with coumarin or furocoumarin content can cause photosensitization and consequently can lead to phototoxic effects such as rashes or blistering. Phototoxicity only occurs with exposure to light or ultraviolet light.

Contraindications and Unusually Toxic Oils

Clinical practice has uncovered possible contraindications for some oils, meaning oils that normally would be unproblematic exert a negative or detrimental effect in the case of an already existing illness. The table on page 49 outlines a variety of known contraindications (according to Dr. Jean Claude Lapraz).[4]

Finally, see the compilation of toxic oils above. Their use is easily avoided as they are not commonly traded on the market.

EXOTIC AND TOXIC OILS

Oil	Active component
Bitter almond	Hydrocyanic acid
Boldo	Ascaridol
Calamus	Asarone
Camphor (yellow)	Saffrol
Goosefoot	Ascaridol
Horseradish	Allyl isothiocyanate
Mugwort	Thujone
Mustard	Allyl isothiocyanate
Pennyroyal	Pulegone
Rue	Methyl nonyl ketone
Sassafras	Safrol
Tansy	Thujone
Thuja	Thujone
Wintergreen	Methyl salicylate
Wormwood	Thujone

The Relationship between Chemical Structure and Effects

Consulting the therapeutic index of an aromatherapy book in order to find an aromamedicinal recommendation for a particular problem can be a discouraging task. In most typical aromatherapy publications, one is confronted with a rather bizarre situation. In one well-known aromatherapy book the section on coughing lists twenty possible oils: anise, benzoin, cajeput, eucalyptus, fir, dwarf pine, pine, marjoram, myrrh, niaouli, peppermint, pepper, rosemary, thyme, juniper, frankincense, hyssop, cinnamon, and cypress. This assortment raises the question: Which oil or oils should actually be used? Other random examples result in similar confusion: The section on insect bites lists basil, savory, cajeput, garlic, lavender, melissa, clove, sage, sassafras, cinnamon, lemon, and onion. Even discounting the fact that both onion and garlic oils are quite problematic to use, the recommendation of essential oils having totally contradictory effects for the same use is perplexing.

Conversely, it is also typical that many different, often contradictory effects are given for a single oil. There are two logical

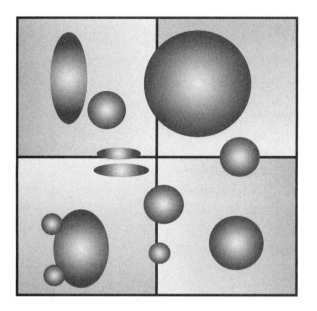

The structure–effect diagram can be thought of as a medicine cabinet whose many containers store substances that treat various symptoms: Essential oils exhibit particular effects depending on their composition.

conclusions: first, the composition of essential oils is so complex that one oil can have many sensible uses; second, despite the broad applicability of essential oils, there is a distinct lack of precision in selecting them. In order to choose the proper oil, more precise criteria are absolutely necessary.

This brings us again to the central point of aromatherapy: taking responsibility for one's own health. The problem cough usually cannot be solved through simply consulting an index and subsequently making a more or less arbitrary selection of oil. The specific conditions in which the cough occurs have to be considered also. In the case of a spasmodic cough, we would choose marjoram oil for the spasmolytic properties of its

ester components. If the cough is an accompanying symptom of a beginning bronchitis, antiviral and expectorant oils, such as cajeput or eucalyptus *(Eucalyptus radiata)* are chosen and the use of decongesting pine oils is delayed until the acute phase is over.

What has been missing in the aromatherapy literature is a simple, conclusive system that connects essential oils and their effects. First, such a system would enable us to recognize the healing effects of an oil based on its position in the system, and, second, to mix essential oils to create optimized synergistic effects.

The classification of the main components of essential oils according to their chemistry and the resulting pharmacological effects constitute the first step toward such a system. With this rough classification and our knowledge of the properties of the terpene molecule we can establish relationships between molecular structure and effect. Molecular structure determines two important qualities: the tendency to either attract or repel electrons, and polarity, which expresses itself, for example, in the degree of affinity to water.

The decisive contribution of Pierre Franchomme to modern aromatherapy was to acknowledge the impact that the tendency to attract or to donate electrons has on the properties of an essential oil component.[1] From experiments involving a great number of essential oils and isolated components, a fascinating picture evolves.

In this experiment essential oils such as melissa or verbena, as well as their main component, citral, produce an electrical current corresponding to electrons given off, while oils such as oregano or thyme, and components such as

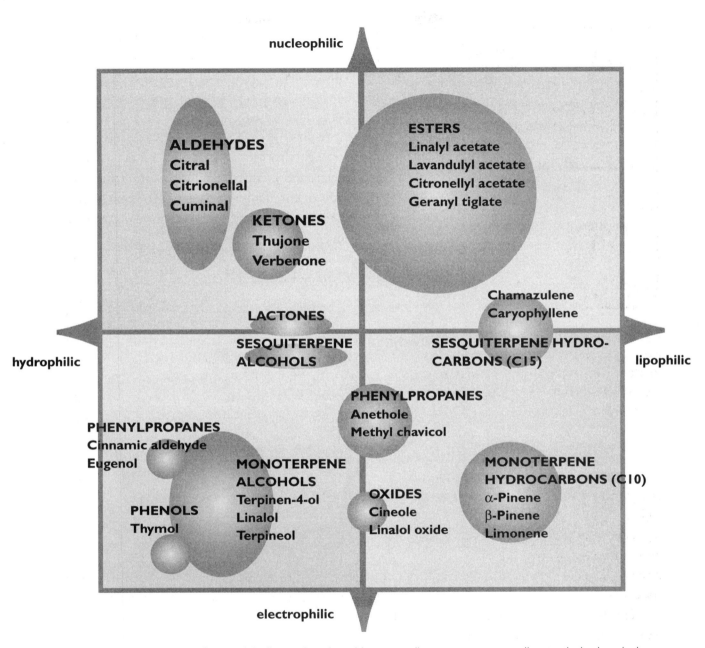

The main components of essential oils can be placed in a coordinate system according to their chemical qualities (their tendency to accept or donate electrons) and their lipophilic or hydrophilic nature.

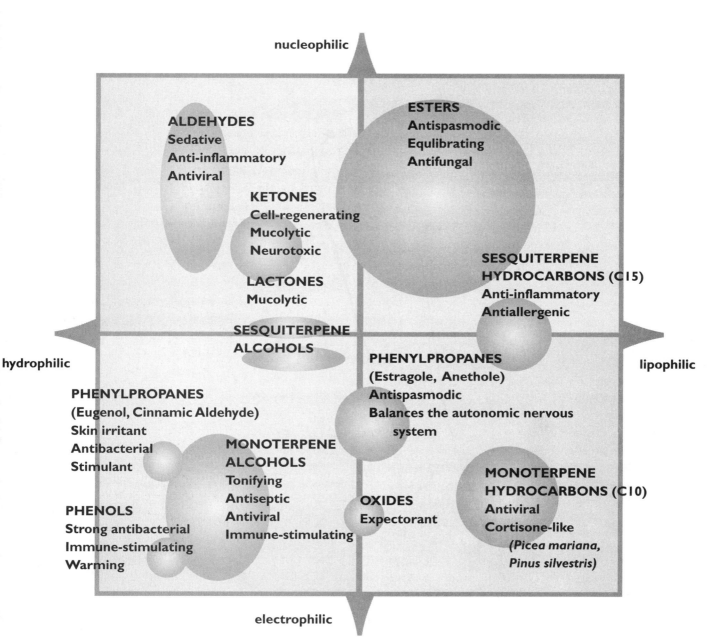

Specific effects can be attributed to the main components of essential oils.

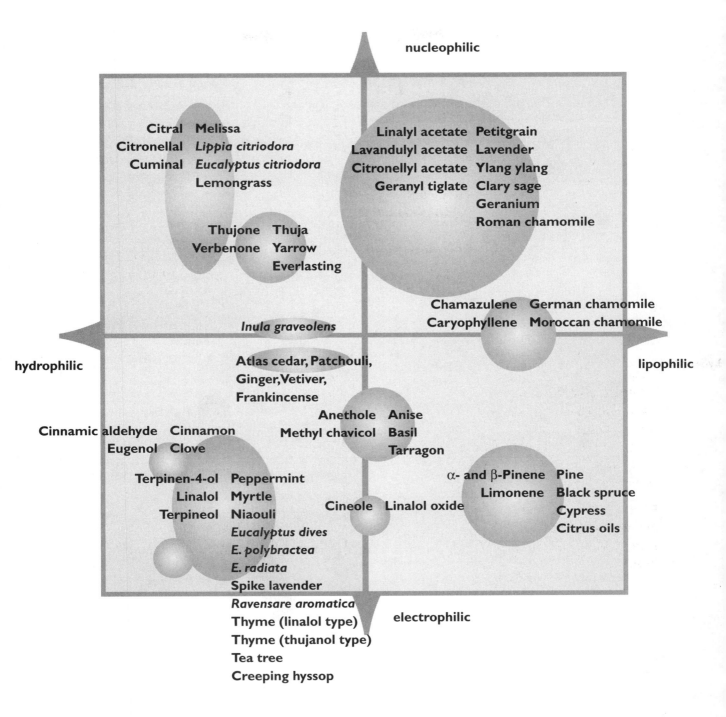

nucleophilic

hydrophilic

lipophilic

electrophilic

Citral **Melissa**	**Linalyl acetate** **Petitgrain**
Citronellal *Lippia citriodora*	**Lavandulyl acetate** **Lavender**
Cuminal *Eucalyptus citriodora*	**Citronellyl acetate** **Ylang ylang**
Lemongrass	**Geranyl tiglate** **Clary sage**
	Geranium
	Roman chamomile

Thujone **Thuja**
Verbenone **Yarrow**
Everlasting

Chamazulene **German chamomile**
Caryophyllene **Moroccan chamomile**

Inula graveolens

Atlas cedar, Patchouli,
Ginger, Vetiver,
Frankincense

Anethole **Anise**
Methyl chavicol **Basil**
Tarragon

Cinnamic aldehyde **Cinnamon**
Eugenol **Clove**

Terpinen-4-ol **Peppermint**
Linalol **Myrtle**
Terpineol **Niaouli**
Eucalyptus dives
E. polybractea
E. radiata
Spike lavender
Ravensare aromatica
Thyme (linalol type)
Thyme (thujanol type)
Tea tree
Creeping hyssop

Cineole **Linalol oxide**

α- and β-Pinene **Pine**
Limonene **Black spruce**
Cypress
Citrus oils

Due to their particular mix of main components essential oils show specific effects. These effects can be utilized to treat specific illnesses.

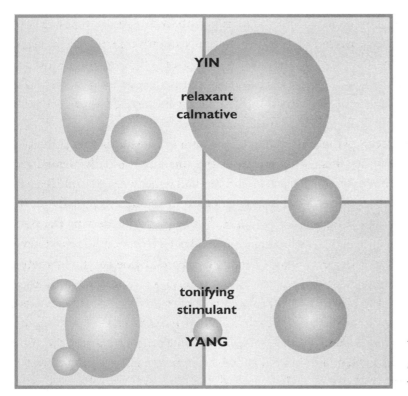

The Chinese principles of *yin* and *yang* are represented in the structure–effect diagram.

carvacrol, thymol, or linalol, produce a current corresponding to the uptake of an electron.

A first distinction of aromatic molecules according to the chemical families they belong to is now possible. Monoterpenes, monoterpene alcohols, and especially phenols display a tendency to take up electrons, along with phenylpropane derivatives and the terpene-oxide cineole.

Electrons are carriers of negative electrical charges. When a molecule picks up an electron, which also means it acquires a negative charge, this in turn creates a positive charge in a neighboring molecule, which causes a certain effect in its surrounding area. In the same way, aromatic molecules which give up electrons influence their surroundings. We observe these processes with the monoterpene ketones, aldehydes, and esters, as well as some unsaturated sesquiterpenes.

Going one step further, the essential oils are now placed in a two-dimensional structure–effect diagram according to the magnitude of the measured current. Oils with the strongest tendency to give up an electron (nucleophiles) are entered on the top of the diagram, those with the tendency to take up electrons (electrophiles) at the bottom. On the horizontal axis, oils are arranged according to their polarity, lipophilic ones to the right and more hydrophilic ones to the left.

What first seemed a rather theoretical exercise has established itself as a useful system for understanding the properties of essential oils in relation to one another. It provides a basis for classifying essential oils according to their chemistry and the resulting effects.

The electrophilic nature of the oils on the

lower side of the structure–effect diagram coincides with a powerful, stimulating character, while oils having a decidedly nucleophilic nature generally exert calming and relaxing influences.

The value of the structure–effect diagram lies in the fact that it allows us to connect a physically measurable parameter with the effects of the oils. Applying the view of Eastern medicine, it is quite possible to recognize the *yin* character of melissa and verbena and, conversely, a definite *yang* character of oregano and cinnamon (see figure on page 56).

This illustrates another aspect of the structure–effect diagram: the basic system can be interpreted and extrapolated in many different ways. Granted, while some conclusions one might deduce could prove truly valuable, others might seem a stretch. But the practical value of making the application of oils simpler and more conclusive is not compromised. It provides a tangible model for approaching complex scientific concepts.

Oil Compositions

The structure–effect diagram proves especially useful when we want to mix oils for a particular purpose. Compositions with especially pronounced synergistic effects result when different oils from one area of the diagram are used, that is, oils that have similar or identically acting main components which mutually increase their effectiveness. The effectiveness of the main components is additionally strengthened by the interaction of the various trace components.

A perfect example of this is the antispasmodic effect of a mixture of equal parts clary sage, Roman chamomile, mandarin petitgrain, and spikenard. The different ester components of these oils mutually improve each other's effect. The sedative effect of spikenard rounds off the cocktail. This mixture is especially effective for neck and shoulder massage and loosens the most persistent tensions.

Another example illustrates this principle: fungus under the toenails is usually beyond the reach of our standard remedy, tea tree oil. Tea tree oil is simply not strong enough to actually get rid of the fungus. But by properly selecting the right combination of oils we can strengthen the desired effect. Mixing two parts thyme (thymol variety), one part oregano, and one part cinnamon, then adding 25 percent of this oil mixture to a base oil, and applying the resultant mixture topically twice daily will eliminate the toughest fungus. (*Caution:* This mixture is designed to be as aggressive as possible, and can therefore only be applied to the toe where skin and nails are hardened and insensitive. Great care should be taken to avoid areas of sensitive, healthy skin, as this mixture can cause major irritation.)

Both of the above examples show that one doesn't have to be a chemist to benefit from the structure–effect principle of oils and their components. It is now easy to understand why a basil oil with a 40 percent linalol content and just a little estragole has a different scent than an exotic basil oil from the Comoro Islands with an 80 percent estragole content. Now we have the means to understand the complex, ever-changing compositions of essential oils and use them effectively.[2]

All in all, there are some interesting developments ahead. We know that using cheap, simplified oils in aromatherapy in no way leads to healing. We know further that the oils' inherent, natural complexity gives them the ability to heal. So, while we profit from the complexities of essential oils, our trusted scientific reductionist instruments cannot sufficiently understand these complexities. What is needed is not simplifying the oils, but discovering new ways to understand their complexities. The structure–effect diagram is a modest beginning, providing a glimpse into the effects of the complex mixtures of essential oil components.

Descriptions of the Oils

The structure–effect diagram of essential oils not only allows us to create optimal combinations, but it offers us a deeper understanding of the effects of both individual oils and their components.

We have now acquired a system of main effects for the twelve most important groups of components of essential oils, and the main effects of a given oil can be represented in a diagram of that form. One example should help to illustrate this: Anise oil has a rather simple makeup. The oil is clearly dominated by its content of 97 percent anethole and the sympatholytic effects of that compound (see structure–effect diagram on page 59).

The structure of niaouli oil is a somewhat different case, since the representation of niaouli oil, its main components being terpene alcohols and the oxide cineole, is more differentiated. Its composition is represented in a diagram (see page 82) in which dark shading depicts the two areas corresponding to these components. We can glean the general character of the oil from the position of the main components, and determine that they are energizing, or yang, oils. Due to the presence of cineole we can expect niaouli to have an expectorant effect as well as antiseptic and strengthening qualities (along with being highly tolerable) due to the presence of terpene alcohols.

There are oils in which active trace or other components induce secondary effects in addition to the main effect. When known, these components are listed along with their effects. In this way, the spectrum of action is represented more precisely.

It is important to realize in any case that essential oils are complex natural mixtures, which can have, aside from the main effects, many different areas of action which cannot be represented in a simplifying diagram.

Under the heading "contraindications" in the following section, the term "physiological dosage" (from Franchomme and Pénoël[3]) refers to an amount of up to a maximum of three drops of pure oil or oil mixture. Here "use with caution" refers to the application of a dose of one or two drops of oil or oil mixture. If, after twelve to twenty-four hours no negative side effects manifest, one can start to use the oil as intended, remaining alert for possible side effects.

Anise *(Pimpinella anisum)*

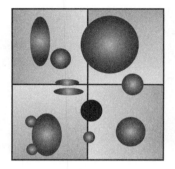

Main component: phenylpropane (anethole)
Main effects: antispasmodic, sedative, stabilizing
Special qualities: estrogen-like, used for amenorrhea
Contraindications: contains ketone; should not be used by children less than 10 years old or pregnant women

The character of anise oil is dominated by the content of 97 percent anethole and its strong calming effect on the nervous system. It acts estrogen-like and can be used for amenorrhea. It minimizes overexcitement and has stabilizing effects following a hangover.

Atlas Cedar *(Cedrus atlanticus)*

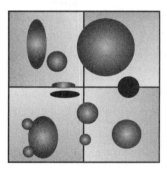

Main component: sesquiterpene-hydrocarbons, -alcohols (atlantol), and -ketones (atlantone)
Main effects: sustained stimulating effects, without irritation
Contraindications: contains ketone; should not be used by children less than 10 years old or pregnant women

Moroccan atlas cedar oil is valued not for any unique medicinal properties, but more for its ability to gently but persistently stimulate circulation and metabolism. It counteracts the storage of excess moisture and fat in tissue, and stimulates their elimination. When combined with certain oils, it is the strongest weapon against cellulite.

Atlas cedar oil is very useful when a composition is desired that has a strong stimulating effect but is not too aggressive or irritating. The stimulating power of atlas cedar oil does not manifest itself as quickly as phenol-containing oils, such as thyme or oregano, but its effects are deeper and longer lasting. With atlas cedar in a certain mixture the desired effect is produced without having to deal with the dominant and somewhat crude aromas of thyme or oregano. The aroma of atlas cedar offers an elegant alternative.

Basil (*Ocimum basilicum*)

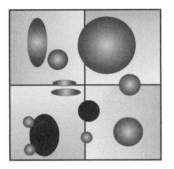

Main components: composition varies; either phenylpropane (methyl chavicol) or terpene alcohols
Main effects: vary according to composition
Contraindications: not for use with small children

The variety of species, subspecies, and chemotypes of basil offer us virtually the entire arsenal of aromatic substances. Basil oil is made in many regions of the world: France, Egypt, Thailand, Nepal, Tanzania, and on the islands in the Indian Ocean. The Comoro Islands and Réunion Island produce a basil oil with a very high estragole content, known as exotic basil oil. An antispasmodic, it has a balancing effect on the autonomic nervous system. The French aromatherapy literature recommends it for Hepatitis A, B, non-A, non-B, and C, as well as yellow fever and tropical viral infections. European basil, in contrast to exotic basil, has a fresher scent due to its higher linalol and lower estragole contents. The European oils are therefore less "harsh," but have less dramatic effects.

Bergamot (*Citrus aurantium* ssp. *bergamia*)

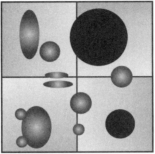

Main components: terpene hydrocarbons, linalyl acetate
Main effects: calming, balancing
Contraindications: phototoxic; should not be applied to skin

Bergamot oil's effects result from the tension between terpene hydrocarbons and esters. Bergamot refreshes, relaxes, and helps relieve insomnia.

Bitter Orange *(Citrus aurantium)*

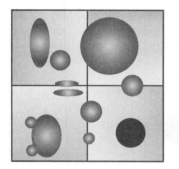

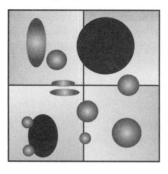

a) rinds: bitter orange
Main components: limonene
Main effects: calms nervousness
Contraindications: phototoxic; should not be applied to skin

c) leaves: petitgrain
Main components: terpene alcohols, linalyl acetate
Main effects: balances the autonomic nervous system
Contraindications: none with physiological dosage

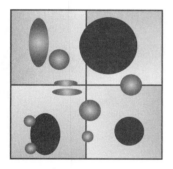

b) flowers: neroli
Main components: terpene hydrocarbons (30%), terpene alcohols (40%), esters (10–20%)
Main effects: relieves anxiety
Contraindications: none with physiological dosage

Citrus aurantium, the tree with three different oils.

Bitter orange, the oil from the rind of the fruit, is used as a calming component in fresh aroma mixtures.

Neroli, the oil from the flowers, is valued for its aroma alone—a drop on the wrist or temples is an effective remedy for anxiety and nervous depression.

The oil from the leaves, petitgrain, also has a stabilizing effect on the nervous system (see illustration above).

Calophyllum (Calophyllum inophyllum)
Main components: not an essential oil, but a fatty oil of varying composition; contains no typical essential oil components
Main effects: stimulates phagocytosis
Contraindications: none when used with caution

The fact that we use the botanical name for this oil, as no common English name is available, indicates that this oil has not been in use long in either conventional medicine or aromatherapy. This oil was introduced to aromamedicine in France, and it is not an essential oil but something of a hybrid, a cross between fatty and aromatic oils—an aromatic fatty oil. It is produced by pressing the fruit of the *Calophyllum inophyllum* tree. It has a blue-green color and an aroma somewhat similar to lovage.

People on the coasts of the Indian Ocean use calophyllum oil as a panacea. It finds its main application as an immune-modulating component in skin-care products, which benefit from its phagocytosis-stimulating qualities. Phagocytosis[4] is a function of our immune system which serves to eliminate unwanted substances. In simpler terms, phagocytosis helps take out the trash.

This oil is recommended in cases of skin conditions accompanied by a buildup of pus. A mixture of equal parts *Ravensare aromatica* and calophyllum oil is an effective treatment for shingles.

Carrot (Daucus carota)

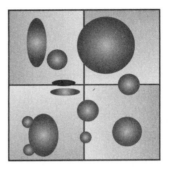

Main components: sesquiterpene hydrocarbons (10%), sesquiterpene alcohol carotol (50%)
Main effects: liver-regenerating
Contraindications: none known

Carrot seed oil is used (because of its sesquiterpene alcohol content—50% carotol) to stimulate regeneration of liver cells. It revitalizes dry, pallid skin.

Chamomile, German and Roman

The discussion of chamomile oils in aromatherapy literature first requires a clear definition of what can truly be considered chamomile. There are only two oils available on the market which can rightfully be called chamomile—German chamomile (*Matricaria recutita*) and Roman chamomile (*Anthemis nobilis*). Other oils are called chamomile because the trade decided at some point that an oil that is blue because it contains some chamazulene sells better when named chamomile. The fact is that oils such as *Ormenis mixta* or *Tanacetum anuum* (see Moroccan chamomile) are not really chamomile oils.

This confusion of terminology is probably due to the fact that, especially in Germany, the word chamomile is connected to so many healing effects that clever business people found the potential for cashing in on these misleading associations quite attractive. If, however, the healing properties of chamomile are desired only true chamomile oils actually distilled from chamomile plants should be used.

German chamomile and Roman chamomile are often described as similar or as more or less identical, which stems from the similarity of the plants. For a meaningful application in aromatherapy it is advantageous to recognize the differences, which are more pronounced in the essential oils of these plants than in their alcohol extracts or teas.

To complicate matters even further, four chemotypes of German chamomile can be distinguished. Of those, the (–)α-bisabolol type performs all the miracles associated with German chamomile. This chemotype has been the most widely researched; therefore, the most knowledge of its pharmacological effects exists. Caution is advised when buying chamomile, as it is mostly the other chemotypes of chamomile which are sold. Any purveyor offering the (–)α-bisabolol type will certainly proudly designate it as such.

German Chamomile (*Matricaria recutita*)

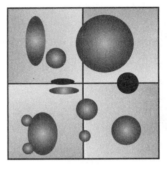

Main components: sesquiterpenes, (–)α-bisabolol, chamazulene
Main effects: anti-inflammatory, antiallergenic
Contraindications: none

The long list of uses ascribed to German chamomile in the literature is impressive and at the same time somewhat discouraging because of the abundance of scientific information.

German chamomile type (–)α-bisabolol is a strongly anti-inflammatory oil, which works the fastest for all types of skin inflammations. Acute conditions, such as burns or allergic rashes react immediately to treatment with German chamomile. The astounding effects of the oil can be observed when treating typical kitchen burns. Simply putting one or two drops of oil on the burn and placing some ice on it will leave no trace of the burn by the next morning. Results with allergic skin reactions are just as impressive.

Naturally, the oil can be used for all other conditions mentioned in the literature. German chamomile is especially user-friendly because it is absolutely nontoxic and can be used in an emergency in its undiluted form.

Roman Chamomile *(Anthemis nobilis)*

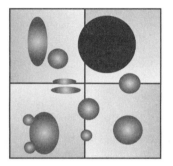

Main components: esters (80%)
Main effects: antispasmodic, calming to the central nervous system; relieves symptoms related to shock
Contraindications: none with physiological dosage

Esters of acids only rarely found in essential oils determine the character of Roman chamomile.

Even in very small concentrations, Roman chamomile, whether alone or in combination with other oils, has a soothing, calming effect. It relieves cramps and spasms and helps relieve shock. In such cases, it is appropriate to massage a few undiluted drops into the solar plexus.

Cinnamon *(Cinnamomum ceylanicum)*

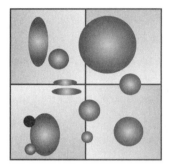

Main components: cinnamic aldehyde
Main effects: general tonic, antiseptic; counteracts enzyme deficiency in digestive tract
Contraindications: caustic to the skin, potentially sensitizing; *not to be used* with children less than 5 years old

Cinnamon bark oil provides ideal, fast-acting relief for infections, enzymatic deficiency in the digestive tract, and bacterial bladder infections.

Caution: Not to be used externally!

Clary Sage *(Salvia sclarea)*

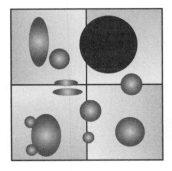

Main components: esters (especially linalyl acetate, 75%)
Main effects: relaxing, spasmolytic
Noteworthy: estrogen-like, used for amenorrhea
Contraindications: mastosis, cancer

Clary sage impresses with its aroma. When applied to the wrists or temples, it is relaxing in a gentle, effective manner. Newcomers to aromatherapy often react to this with a light euphoria and giddiness. Robert Tisserand was the first aromatherapist to describe the occurrence of these euphoric effects during massage. This oil has intense effects on some individuals and more moderate effects on others. Through its sclareol content clary sage has an estrogen-like quality and is used to ease premenstrual syndrome.

Clove *(Eugenia caryophyllata)*

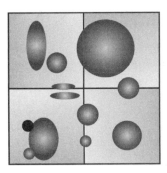

Main components: eugenol (80%)
Main effects: antiseptic, having a broad spectrum of action against bacteria; antiviral, strengthening
Contraindications: irritating to the skin, potentially sensitizing. External use only after a negative allergy test. Use only in a highly diluted solution (maximum 1 drop per 20-milliliter solution).

Clove bud oil is used in dentistry and has a broad spectrum of action against bacteria. In aromatherapy it is used for viral hepatitis, amebiasis, tuberculosis, and asthenia. Clove bud oil can be sensitizing.

Coriander *(Coriandrum sativum)*

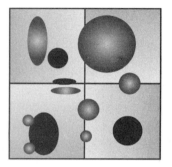

Main components: terpene alcohols (up to 80%, primarily linalol)
Main effects: strengthening; promotes digestion; can cause a mild feeling of euphoria
Noteworthy: coumarin and furocoumarin
Contraindications: none known

Because of the high linalol content, this oil is tonifying and strengthening. In addition, a series of coumarin compounds together with linalol provides a mild euphoric effect.

Cypress *(Cupressus sempervirens)*

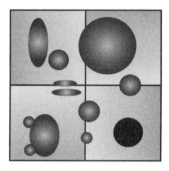

Main components: terpene hydrocarbons (70%)
Main effects: decongesting for veins and lymphs, antibiotic
Noteworthy: active sesquiterpene and diterpene alcohols
Contraindications: mastosis

In all of aromatherapy there is perhaps no oil more effective than cypress oil to counteract an infection of either the throat, nose, or bronchi in its early phase. Used at the very first signs of sore throat, it is typically sufficient to arrest the process and prevent the development of subsequent bronchitis or a cold.

This application is simple: one drop is taken as soon as scratchiness or soreness in the throat point to a beginning infection. As the admittedly disagreeable turpentine taste develops in the mouth, any soreness in the throat will become overshadowed by this pervasive taste. After a few minutes, the taste changes, taking on a relatively pleasing character. As the sore throat sensation returns, another drop of cypress oil is taken. This procedure is repeated until one gets somewhat used to the taste. After the third, fourth, or fifth application, the soreness typically will not return. Without the prompt of the sore throat, one generally forgets to continue taking cypress oil, which is the desired, self-regulating effect.

Eucalyptus (*Eucalyptus* spec.)

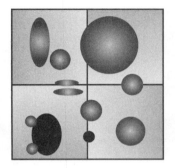

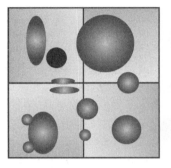

a) *Eucalyptus radiata*
Main components: terpene alcohols, cineole
Main effects: expectorant, antiviral
Contraindications: none known

The composition of this oil is such that it could be considered an aromatherapist's "designer oil." Together with its attractive fragrance and low price this is the number one all-purpose eucalptus oil. The combination of terpene alcohols and cineole is highly effective in treating coughing, sniffles, and a hoarse, scratchy throat. It also contains 3 to 4 percent aldehydes (including neral and geraniol), which lend this oil an especially broad spectrum of action (antiviral, expectorant, anti-inflammatory), as well as its exceptionally pleasant aroma.

b) *Eucalyptus dives*
Main components: terpene hydrocarbons
   (30%), piperitone (approximately 50%)
Main effects: mucolytic
Contraindications: contains ketone; not to
   be used by children less than 10 years old
   or pregnant women

With this oil, it is mainly the piperitone chemotype that is of interest. It is distinguished by a content of approximately 50 percent of this relatively harmless ketone, which makes it a highly effective, reasonably priced, mucolytic agent for bronchitis. Mix with *Eucalyptus radiata* to enhance and diversify its effects.

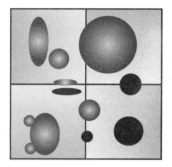

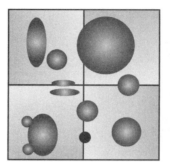

c) *Eucalyptus globulus*
Main components: up to 75% terpene
hydrocarbons, cineole, sesquiterpenes, and
alcohols
Main effects: expectorant
Contraindications: not to be used with small
children

Eucalyptus globulus is the most well-known euca-lyptus variety. This oil has a unique, fresh scent which is enhanced by the presence of sesquiter-penes and various aldehydes. As with *Eucalyptus radiata*, *E. globulus* is a good expectorant and is suitable for treating cold symptoms.

d) *Eucalyptus polybractea*
Main components: terpene oxide (cineole)
Main effects: expectorant
Contraindications: none when used with
caution

Like other types of eucalyptus oils, *Eucalyptus polybractea* is also an effective expectorant. It is especially suited for improving room air with a diffusor.

Everlasting *(Helichrysum italicum)*

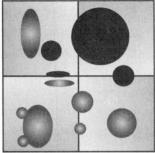

Main components: esters (neryl acetate, 40–50%), sesquiterpene hydrocarbons (30%)
Main effects: anti-inflammatory, cell-regenerating
Noteworthy: up to 10% diketones
Contraindications: safe despite ketone content

The high content of anti-inflammatory, calming sesquiterpene hydrocarbons is complimented by the presence of approximately 40 percent spasmolytic esters and approximately 8 percent regenerative diketones (found only in everlasting). The pain-reducing, analgesic, and regenerative effect of everlasting is unique: if applied in time, it prevents hemorrhaging. It is also very effective for joint pain associated with rheumatoid arthritis.

Frankincense *(Boswellia carteri)*

Main components: terpene and sesquiterpene hydrocarbons
Main effects: anti-asthmatic, strengthens the immune system
Contraindications: none known

Frankincense consists primarily of terpene hydrocarbons, in addition to small concentrations of complex molecules with two functional groups. This oil is used for weakened immune system, asthma, and depression.

Geranium *(Pelargonium odorantissimum)*

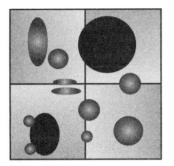

Main components: terpene alcohols (60–68%), esters (20–33%)
Main effects: general tonic, fungicide
Contraindications: none

Geranium is produced in many different countries and consequently offered in different compositions with varying properties. Different distillation methods explain the variety of colors of geranium oil, ranging from brownish yellow to light green. The scent of geranium oil enjoys broad popularity, due to its citronellol content, which it shares with rose oil. This alcohol (citronellol) and a wide spectrum of esters lend geranium oil its pleasant character. The tonifying effect of the terpene alcohol combined with the soothing influence of the esters are responsible for the fact that geranium oil is perceived differently by each individual. One person will perceive it as an antiseptic, another as a calmative, and a third as a stimulant.

Despite—or perhaps because of—this versatile character, geranium oil is an excellent foundation for massage and body oils. Because of its ester content, geranium oil is also remarkably effective against *Candida albicans* and other fungi, as well as being especially valuable in skin care and holistic hygiene.

Interestingly, the antimycotic effect of geranium is not linked—as is the case with many other oils—to an antibacterial effect; this means geranium acts against yeasts without affecting bacterial flora. In addition, geranium stops bleeding, stimulates the functions of the liver and pancreas, and, applied topically, soothes pain in the breasts before and during menstruation (10 milliliters geranium oil with 100 milliliters base oil).

Green Myrtle *(Myrtus communis)*

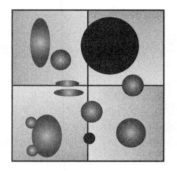

Main components: monoterpene oxide
(cineole)
Main effects: expectorant
Noteworthy: Esters, aldehydes, and lactones
make this oil suitable for treating tension
and insomnia
Contraindications: none

The oil of *Myrtus communis* varies in composition depending on whether it comes from the northern or southern shores of the Mediterranean. North African myrtle generally has a reddish or reddish brown color and contains the ester myrtenyl acetate. The Corsican variety of *Myrtus communis* has a brilliant green color and a high 1,8-cineole content. The green Corsican oil is produced exclusively for the aromatherapy market. There are no industrial uses. It is available at a somewhat high but fair cost in small quantities.

If it is inhaled directly, green myrtle has an astounding relaxing effect. It is also used as a gentle, nonirritating component in skin-care mixtures, where it displays its regenerating, astringent, and anti-allergenic effects best. In addition, it imparts them with a truly elegant scent.

This oil is especially useful for treating hay fever (see page 112), especially for patients who have been using *Eucalyptus radiata* or various needle oils fairly often and need a change of scent or effects.

Myrtle Hydrosol (myrtle water)

Myrtle water is the most useful of all the essential oil hydrosols as it covers an area otherwise inaccessible to aromatherapy: the eyes. Essential oils do not mix with the watery environment of the eyes, and they also irritate them. Consequently, irritations of the eyes, caused by accidental contact with an essential oil, are best taken care of by imbuing a piece of cloth or papertowel with a fatty oil, such as sesame or olive oil, and wiping it over the closed eyelids. The fatty oil will draw the lipophilic essential oil from the eye more effectively than rinsing the eye with water or other similar measures.

Myrtle water is especially suited for treating all forms of inflammatory processes in the eyes, by spraying it directly on the eyelid or in the eye. The novice user will spray on closed eyes, and try to blink a little bit. Repeated spraying will be effective against conjunctivitis, allergic reactions, and all inflammations of the eye.

Myrtle water should not be used after the expiration date provided by the manufacturer.

Greenland Moss (*Ledum grönlandicum*)

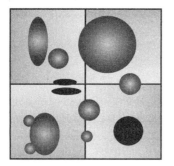

Main components: terpene hydrocarbons
Main effects: purifying; detoxifies the liver
Special qualities: sesquiterpene-ketones,
  germacrone
Contraindications: none

This oil contains active sesquiterpene-ketones. It is used to stimulate regeneration of the liver, and it detoxifies the liver and kidneys.

Creeping Hyssop (*Hyssopus officinalis* var. *decumbens*)

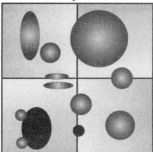

Main components: terpene alcohols
Main effects: strong antiviral effects, anti-
  asthmatic, antidepressant
Noteworthy: trans-linalol oxide
Contraindications: none known

Creeping hyssop oil (*Hyssopus officinalis* var. *decumbens*) has perhaps the strongest antiviral effects and is therefore especially suitable for treating herpes and fever blisters. Combined with Khella (*Ammi visnaga*), it is used to prevent asthma attacks. Used for nervous depression it has an uplifting effect and helps an individual to lighten up.

Inula graveolens

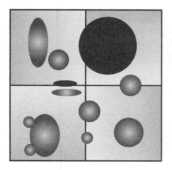

Main components: esters (bornyl acetate, 50%)
Main effects: mucolytic, heart tonic
Special qualities: sesquiterpene lactones make it a most powerful mucolytic
Contraindications: none when used with caution

Inula graveolens is generally only found on the French aromatherapy market, and even then at a very high price and only in years with a very good harvest.

Despite its uncertain availability, it is recommended for all bronchitis conditions, for which its usefulness cannot be overestimated. It is so effective that a family of four using it correctly will certainly not need more than 5 milliliters in one year.

What makes this oil so unusual? In brief, it is the strongest mucolytic to be found in aromatherapy.

Of this brilliant green oil only the main components are known. It contains traces of lactones which, although not yet identified, seem to be pharmacologically very active. This oil is most effective when it comes to loosening mucus. The effect is so pronounced that it occurs even at concentrations below odor threshold.

The best method of use is in a diffusor at night, with the output of the diffusor set at the lowest possible level. Otherwise, one can simply put a drop of oil on a pillow.

This oil is most effective against all catarrhal illnesses of the upper respiratory tract (throat, nose), against chronic bronchitis, and also against spasmodic conditions.

Khella *(Ammi visnaga)*

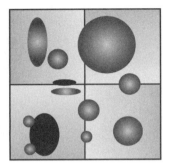

Main components: terpenes, terpene alcohols (borneol, linalol)
Main effects: dilates coronary blood vessels; with asthma and hay fever, it relieves spasms in the smooth muscle tissue of the bronchi
Noteworthy: contains coumarin and related compounds (visnadin, khellin)
Contraindications: phototoxic; not to be used on the skin

This oil has a dilating effect, especially on the coronary blood vessels, the bronchi, and the urinary tract. It is used for asthma and gallbladder and kidney colics.

Laurel *(Laurus nobilis)*

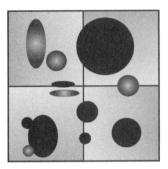

Main components: cineole, esters, terpene alcohols, eugenol
Main effects: anti-infective, equilibrates the autonomic nervous system
Contraindications: none known; should be used sparingly for external applications to avoid potential sensitization

The composition of bay laurel, especially European grown, is multifaceted. Bay laurel contains elements of nearly all of the described twelve main chemical groups, which explains the wide spectrum of positive effects. Long perceived as powerful, laurel is a symbol of victory throughout Greek and Roman mythology.

There are a number of varieties of the essential oil of bay laurel. The oils from North Africa have an aroma reminiscent of eucalyptus due to their high cineole content. These oils are only of secondary importance in aromatherapy. The oils produced in Italy, France, and the former Yugoslavia have a lower cineole content (approximately 35 percent) and a more refined aroma reminiscent of the bay leaf used in cooking. These delicately scented oils from the northern Mediterranean are preferred for aromatherapy use.

Although there are no scientific studies on

the medicinal effects of bay laurel, its positive effects on the lymphatic system are undeniable. Rubbing a few drops of bay laurel on swollen lymph nodes will produce an immediately noticeable relieving effect. The positive and pleasant effect of this oil is so distinct and strong that one application will normally suffice to convince the most hardened skeptic to use it.

A variation of this application is to use bay laurel oil in the sauna. Rubbing a few drops into the lymph nodes and solar plexus after some time has been spent in the sauna will quickly bring on its gentle, pleasant effects on the skin. The resulting stimulation is gentle but strengthening.

Caution: Frequent use of bay laurel oil on the skin over a longer period of time (e.g., longer than three weeks) can result in sensitization and irritability because of its content of sesquiterpene lactones. As with anything, a happy medium is the key to success. For a healthy body, one application weekly is an effective preventive measure. During flu season it can be applied more frequently. After the acute phase of the illness is over it is advisable to take a break from using bay laurel.

Lavender (*Lavandula angustifolia*)

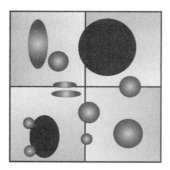

Main components: linalol and linalyl acetate
Main effects: balancing, relieves tension, relieves pain
Contraindications: none with physiological dosage

Lavender comes in many forms. Depending on origin and the altitude at which it is grown, its composition varies greatly. In general, French lavenders are characterized by a high ester content, for which they are esteemed by perfumers worldwide. It has therefore become a usual but undesirable practice to add the ester linalyl acetate to the oil to reach a level of 40 percent.

Actually, one should always have a bottle of lavender oil close at hand as it works wonders for burns. It is also highly effective for relieving itching insect bites, heals small cuts (such as paper cuts), and generally keeps the skin in healthy balance. Interestingly, lavender also normalizes blood sugar output by the liver. One or two drops taken about fifteen minutes before a meal will noticeably reduce the appetite.

The oil that is produced in Croatia and known as lavender, but which is actually produced from a local hybrid (*Lavandula hybrida*, Burdrorka), is also effective for the purposes of aromatherapy. This oil contains significant amounts of borneol and terpinen-4-ol and has stronger antiseptic qualities than the French oil. It is suitable for treating infected hair follicles and other minor skin conditions (pimples, blackheads, and light forms of acne).

When it comes to blending oils, lavender has a special quality. It harmonizes scents of different origins. Adding a small amount of lavender to a mixture will make the blend round and harmonious.

Lemon *(Citrus limon)*

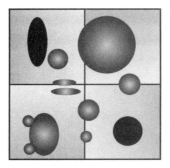

Main components: terpene hydrocarbons
Main effects: antiseptic, stimulates digestion, prevents contagious illnesses, such as colds and flu
Noteworthy: coumarin
Contraindications: phototoxic; *do not* apply to the skin.

This oil with the refreshing scent stimulates the liver, has a gentle, calming effect (despite its high terpene hydrocarbon content), and is perhaps the most effective oil for disinfecting room air using a diffusor.

Lemon Verbena *(Lippia citriodora)*

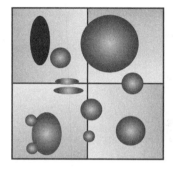

Main components: geraniol, neral (about 40% combined)
Main effects: anti-inflammatory, calming, antidepressant
Special qualities: complex composition, many special effects (see below)
Contraindications: none with physiological dosage; contains traces of furocoumarin; can have photosensitizing effects on the skin

Lemon verbena's scent is gentler and more pleasant than that of all other oils with a high citral content. It works strongly on the psycho-hormonal level. It is strongly anti-inflammatory and calming and used to treat depression. Aromamedicine uses this oil as a supplemental treatment for malaria, multiple sclerosis, and Hodgkin's disease.

Mandarin *(Citrus reticulata)*

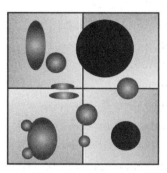

Main components: terpene hydrocarbons, especially limonene
Main effects: relieves anxiety
Noteworthy: esters of anthranilic acid
Contraindications: can be phototoxic to the skin

The scent of mandarin is as sweet as candy. The presence of the highly sedative anthranilic acid ester makes this oil the first choice for use with children suffering from anxiety, nervousness, or stress. Mandarin oil can be taken internally and can be used to freshen indoor air.

Tangerine oil has a scent very similar to that of mandarin, but it contains no anthranilic acid ester and has no sedative effects. Fluoresce—observable with mandarin oil—is not present.

Mandarin Petitgrain (*Citrus reticulata*)

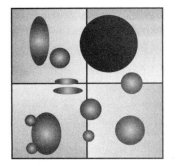

Main components: esters (methyl anthranilate)
Main effects: strongly relaxing
Contraindications: none known

This oil from the leaves of the mandarin tree is above all stress-relieving. It is so effective that even small amounts (1 to 5 percent in a mixture) added to other calming oils will drastically strengthen the sedative effect of the composition.

Marjoram (*Origanum majorana*)

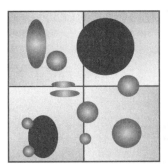

Main components: terpene alcohol (terpinen-4-ol), terpene esters
Main effects: anti-infective, spasmolytic
Noteworthy: effective against whooping cough
Contraindications: none with physiological dosage

Marjoram oil is unique in its composition of relaxing, spasmolytic esters with a significant 25 percent content of terpinen-4-ol. This is the same alcohol that renders tea tree oil such an effective antiseptic.

The uses of marjoram extend from replacing tea tree oil—if one should tire of tea tree's strong scent—to other uses for which its special combination of properties makes it most effective. For example, it is used for whooping cough (see page 110) and acute bronchitis with accompanying cough, in which the spasmolytic effect is of special value. Marjoram oil is either taken internally or applied to the skin.

Caution: In addition to the marjoram (*Origanum majorana*) oil discussed above, different oil from another plant species, *Thymus mastichina,* is often sold under the names "marjoram," "wild marjoram," or "Spanish marjoram." This oil should *not be confused* with the true marjoram oil described here, as its composition and effects are different.

Mastic *(Pistacius lentiscus)*

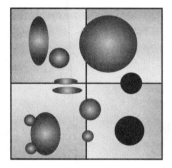

Main components: terpene- and
sesquiterpene-hydrocarbons
Main effects: decongesting for veins, lymph,
etc.
Contraindications: none known

Mastic oil is distilled from the resin of the mastic tree, predominately on the island of Crete. In aromatherapy it is valued for its vasoconstrictive action, especially in the treatment of varicose veins.

May Chang *(Litsea cubeba)*

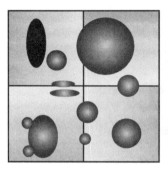

Main components: terpene aldehydes
(geranial and neral, together composing
approximately 75%)
Main effects: calming, anti-inflammatory
Contraindications: none when used with
caution

Litsea cubeba is valued for its high content of citral, due to which it normally is used only in combination with other oils. Its refreshing scent makes it perfect for giving a composition a brighter scent. When the antiviral and regenerating qualities of citral are needed, this oil is a cost-effective solution.

Melissa (*Melissa officinalis*)

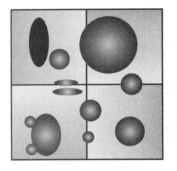

Main components: terpene aldehydes (neral, geranial)
Main effects: relieves depression, nervous weakness, and insomnia
Contraindications: none with physiological dosage

The way in which melissa oil combines an excellent antiviral component with a soothing but pervasive sedative power is difficult to imagine; it has to be experienced. In its complexity, power, and gentleness, melissa oil perfectly illustrates how nature time after time works better than one-dimensional synthetic medicines.

Melissa oil appears to be one of the strongest antiviral agents available in aromatherapy. With only a few topical applications a herpes outbreak can be ended and the blisters dried up.

Rubbing a trace of the oil on the temples will ease a headache. The sedative and anti-inflammatory effect of this oil can be utilized best in many external applications (see page 102).

Note: It is advisable to use the oil for these purposes in very low concentrations. For this, melissa is mixed with a base oil in a ratio of 1:100. An even smaller portion of melissa will still have excellent results.

Moroccan Chamomile (*Tanacetum annuum*)

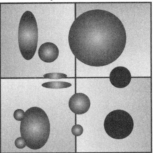

Main components: monoterpenes (limonene), sesquiterpenes (azulene)
Main effects: anti-inflammatory (especially on the skin), anti-allergenic, anti-asthmatic
Contraindications: none known

This oil is striking not only for its blue color—due to a high azulene content—but also because of its sweet, aromatic scent. Moroccan chamomile is an obligatory component for any mixture used for burns or sunburns, or otherwise inflamed or damaged skin. It is also a must for ameliorating allergic reactions. It is most effective applied externally or by inhalation by adding a few drops to 5 or 10 milliliters of a mixture (see page 116).

Moroccan Thyme *(Thymus satureioides)*

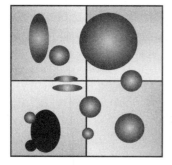

Myrrh *(Commiphora molmol)*

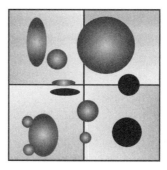

Main components: terpene alcohols (borneol, phenol, carvacrol)
Main effects: strengthening
Noteworthy: especially effective against chronic infections and in strengthening a weakened immune system
Contraindications: can cause mild skin irritation

The only readily available oil with a distinctively high content of borneol, Moroccan thyme oil is best suited for treating chronic infections and autoimmune conditions. It relieves arthrosis and counteracts general asthenia.

Main components: terpene hydrocarbons, sesquiterpenes
Main effects: anti-inflammatory, antiviral
Noteworthy: sesquiterpene ether
Contraindications: none known

Myrrh has antiviral and anti-inflammatory properties. It is primarily used for diarrhea, but also as a mouthwash in dental care.

Niaouli (*Melaleuca quinquenervia viridiflora*, MQV)

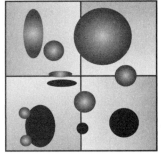

Main components: terpene hydrocarbons, terpene alcohols, sesquiterpene alcohols, terpene oxide (cineole)
Main effects: expectorant, strengthening
Contraindications: none known; hormone-like effects. Children less than 10 years old and pregnant women should *use with caution*.

Niaouli comes from New Caledonia and Madagascar. The New Caledonian oil used to be "cut" and had a relatively uniform odor. Madagascar oil has proven itself for aromatherapy use. To differentiate between the two the abbreviation MQV (for the botanical name *Melaleuca quinquenervia viridiflora*) was often used by Pierre Franchomme and became something of a trade name for that oil. Niaouli oil is as complex in its composition as it is in its uses.

The persistence of this tree is currently vexing United States environmentalists. Once it has taken root, the tree refuses to go away. This has happened in southern Florida, where this species has spread unchecked for several years. Clearing the trees by cutting provides no solution, as even stumps of felled trees simply grow back. As if that were not enough, allergists have recognized the pollen of niaouli trees as a powerful allergen. The spread of this tree is considered responsible for a great increase of allergic conditions in Florida.

These facts point to the most important qualities of niaouli oil. It is anti-allergenic and strengthening and yet another example of the phenomenon that an agent that causes a condition can also heal it. Niaouli oil is one of the most important anti-allergenics in the aromatherapy arsenal.

Niaouli oil also has the ability to tighten tissue and is used for hemorrhoids. The oil is effective for specific and general skin problems and can be used undiluted without risk.

In some cases, however, it may cause skin irritation; then it should be substituted with tea tree oil, or mixed with tea tree or lavender (in a ratio of 1:1 to 1:4). Niaouli is nontoxic and can be used liberally. One of the fastest-acting and most effective applications of niaouli is to apply anywhere between 5 and 20 drops to the whole body during the morning shower. This procedure will become entirely holistic if a loofah glove is used and the oil is worked into the skin along the energy meridians. This application is refreshing and invigorating and is especially recommended in flu season, as it stimulates the defense mechanisms of the body.

Rubbing niaouli on the gums strengthens them, diminishing inflammation, and the oil's antiseptic qualities protect the mouth and throat. Niaouli can also be used on dental floss to cleanse the spaces between the teeth.

Because niaouli has some estrogen-like characteristics, common sense and alertness are advised when hormonal imbalances are present.

Oregano *(Origanum vulgaris)*

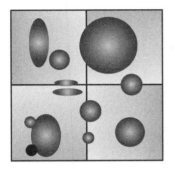

Main components: phenols (carvacrol)
Main effects: antibacterial, stimulating
Contraindications: not to be used on the
skin (dermocaustic)

In oregano oils, we encounter high concentrations of the antiseptic and stimulating phenol carvacol, in combination with stimulating terpene hydrocarbons. A certain ketone and sesquiterpene content (approximately 6 percent caryophyllene) balances the extreme effects of phenol.

When it comes to combating bacterial infections, oregano is aromatherapy's heavy artillery. It also has stimulating qualities. Because its phenols can cause varying degrees of skin irritation, it recommends itself for internal use. Ideally oregano oil is taken in a carrier oil, such as sunflower. The amount of oregano oil should be about 50 milligrams per application.

Oregano oil is well suited for treating acute bacterial infections of the gastrointestinal tract and the bronchi. When a strong response to a bacterial infection is needed, taking up to ten dosages of 50 milligrams of oregano (equivalent to 1–2 drops per application or $\frac{1}{2}$ gram in total per day) will do the trick. Thyme and mountain savory oils have similar effects due to their similar compositions.

In general, use of oregano oil should be limited to treating acute conditions. The French aromamedical literature advises that the long-term use of this oil, or generally oils with a high phenol content, can lead to undesirable changes in the liver metabolism.

Palmarosa (*Cymbopogon martini*)

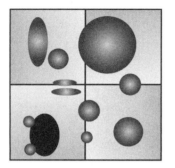

Main components: terpene alcohol (geraniol)
Main effects: effective against bacterial and
viral illnesses of throat and lungs
Contraindications: none with physiological
dosage

One could say that this oil is the dream of every
aromatherapy enthusiast. It is inexpensive and
combines an impressive variety of desirable qualities. It is effective against viruses, yet it is mild
and nontoxic, and has a very attractive scent.
This oil is perfect as a central, reasonably priced
component for antiseptic skin-care compositions.

Patchouli (*Pogostemon cablin*)

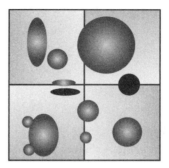

Main components: sesquiterpenes, sesquiter-
pene alcohols
Main effects: vein tonic
Contraindications: none known

Patchouli—the scent of the hippie generation.
Its scent certainly is the most prominent feature
of this oil. But, used externally, it is also a good
tonic for veins.

Peppermint *(Mentha piperita)*

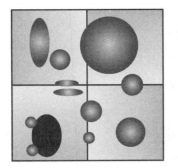

Main components: menthol, menthone
Main effects: stimulating, strengthening
Contraindications: topical applications need
to be limited to small areas (for example,
on the forehead or temples); *not to be used*
on infants less thatn 30 months old.

For the aromatherapy user, peppermint oil is as indispensable as it is problematic: indispensable due to its healing properties; problematic due to the many different qualities and compositions in which it is offered.

Peppermint oil is produced on an industrial scale in the United States and in China, mainly for the production of menthol. Most oils produced in the U.S. are standardized blends of different oils of varying qualities from regions such as the Midwest and the Pacific Northwest.

The oils produced in England or France are the most suitable for use in aromatherapy, as they are produced for this purpose and are generally not doctored or minimally doctored. The price differential between generic oils produced for the world market and genuine oils produced for aromatherapy is significant.

Peppermint oil should be a part of every traveler's first-aid kit. A drop works wonders for motion sickness or general nausea. In addition, medical research has found that peppermint is effective for irritable colon. French aromamedicine recommends peppermint oil for general asthemia as it strengthens and regenerates the liver.

Peppermint oil is also an appropriate means for adding some zest to a bland mixture of oils. For this, a concentration of between .25 percent and .50 percent is sufficient. Naturally, one can experiment individually with more or less, but the strongest effects normally are achieved when peppermint oil is used sparingly.

Pine *(Pinus pinaster)*

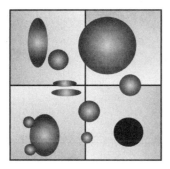

Main components: terpene hydrocarbons
Main effects: applied topically as a disinfectant,
or in a diffusor used as an air freshener
Contraindications: not for internal use

An inexpensive oil for use in a diffusor, pine oil has a strong antiseptic effect for bronchial illnesses. The high monoterpene hydrocarbon content is characteristic of needle oils. Sesquiterpene hydrocarbons and sesquiterpene alcohols round off its effects.

Ravensare *(Ravensare aromatica)*

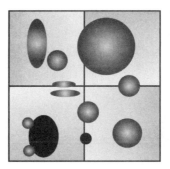

Main components: terpene alcohols, terpene
oxides (cineole)
Main effects: expectorant, antiviral
Contraindications: none known; well tolerated on the skin

An oil used in French aromatherapy known by the name of *ravensare* really comes from the leaves of *Cinnamomum camphora*. Despite the confusion of names its chemical composition and identity are well defined.

Ravensare oil's effectiveness appears to stem from the interaction between cineole and α-terpineol. It is light and not dissimilar to *Eucalyptus radiata*. It is used primarily to treat viral conditions.

In addition to its strong antiviral effects, ravensare is also valued as an excellent nerve tonic. It works small wonders with acute cases of the flu, raising overall energy and creating an optimistic mood. Ravensare is best suited for treating mononucleosis and for relieving insomnia. Its most notable use is in the treatment of shingles in conjunction with *Calophyllum inophyllum*. For the treatment of acute flu, ravensare is best taken internally (1 drop every 2 hours for acute flu) and/or applied externally.

Rose (*Rosa damascena*)

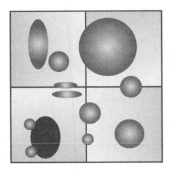

Main components: terpene alcohols (citronellol), approximately 50%, paraffin (as in waxes)
Main effects: nerve tonic
Contraindications: none known

The unfortunately very expensive rose oil is best used for its fragrance. The scent alone has uplifting and tonifying effects and stabilizes the nervous system.

Rosemary (*Rosmarinus officinalis*)

In aromatherapy, rosemary is a problem oil. Hardly any other oil is so routinely adulterated and diluted. Diverse scientific articles point to contradictory results which can only be explained by widespread adulteration. According to the estimates of a group of German experts, the cost of manufacturing rosemary oil is at least 200–300 German Marks (about U.S. $112.00–170.00) per kilogram. How this relates to the usual wholesale price of $30.00 to $50.00 remains unexplained. When buying this oil, close attention must be paid to its source, and only products whose origins can be traced back to the manufacturer should be accepted. Quality can only be provided by producers who make the oil exclusively for the aromatherapy market, and whose oils will command the appropriate price. A small number of producers of rosemary oils are currently located in Croatia and Corsica.

Three chemotypes of rosemary oil are recognized. They are outlined below.

Rosemary—camphor type (Spain and Croatia)

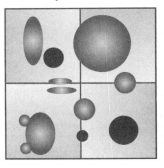

Main components: terpene ketone (camphor), terpene oxide (cineole), terpene hydrocarbons
Main effects: neuromuscular, stimulating for asthenia, relieves tension

Contraindications: contains ketone; *not to be used* by children less than 10 years old or pregnant women

An oil for many uses, especially for muscles and nerves, this type is especially suitable for muscle pain and cramps. In small dosage it relieves nervous tension; in higher dosage it counteracts exhaustion. Expectedly, rosemary supports the digestive system: it stimulates the production of bile.

Rosemary—cineole type (North Africa)

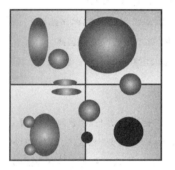

Main components: cineole, terpene hydrocarbons
Main effects: stimulating, promotes digestion
Contraindications: none with physiological dosage

Especially suited for catarrhal conditions and as a component for diffusor mixtures.

Rosemary—verbenone type (Corsica)

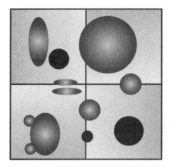

Main components: ketones (verbenone), cineole, terpene hydrocarbons
Main effects: mucolytic, promotes digestion, cell-regenerating (skin care)
Contraindications: ketone content. Children less than 10 years old and pregnant women should use with caution.

An aromatherapy classic, this oil's regenerating qualities and the way it is tolerated by the skin make it essential for skin care. It is especially effective as the beginning mucolytic treatment of bronchial and cold conditions.

Sage (*Salvia officinalis*)

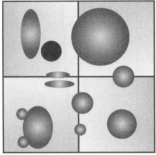

Main components: high concentration of ketones (up to 70%), primarily thujone

Main effects: strengthening, promotes digestion, estrogen-like

Noteworthy: broad spectrum of action, but difficult to categorize due to varying compositions

Contraindications: high ketone content; *not to be used* by children less than 10 years old or pregnant women

The main ingredient of sage oil is thujone (20–70 percent). Besides that it contains a great number of active molecules which provide a diverse range of complex effects. It is effective against *Staphylococcus aureus* and bacteria of the genus *Streptococcus* and has an antiviral effect. Sage is also used to stimulate bile production.

Spike Lavender (*Lavandula latifolia*)

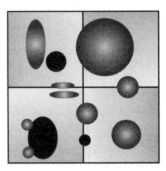

Main components: cineole, terpene alcohols, terpene ketone (camphor)

Main effects: expectorant, antiviral

Contraindications: depends on camphor content; small children and pregnant women should use only with extreme caution

Spike lavender is a practical oil: while the scent is not as delicate as that of true lavender, its camphor and cineole content make spike lavender very useful for colds. It is most effective when used together with the linalol chemotype of thyme as an expectorant–antiviral mixture to be massaged into the skin (see page 97). For skin care, this oil can be used as a mild but effective antiseptic.

Spikenard (Nardostachys jatamansi)

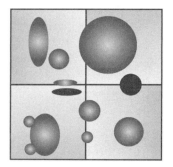

Main components: sesquiterpenes, sesquiterpene alcohols, and sesquiterpene ketones
Main effects: sedative
Contraindications: none known

This oil consists primarily of sedative components. It contains only sesquiterpenoids, such as valeranol, valerenal, and especially valeranone, which are responsible for the sedative effect.

The external application of the oil, rubbed over the heart or the solar plexus, provides the desired sedative effect. This oil has a distinct affinity to the skin, and is one of the few oils which has any effect against dandruff.

Spruce (Picea mariana)

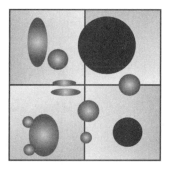

Main components: terpene hydrocarbons and esters (bornyl acetate)
Main effects: general strengthening for asthenic conditions
Contraindications: none with physiological dosage

Spruce oil restores depleted adrenal glands. Combined with *Pinus silvestris* and applied externally over the kidney area it will reenergize. Spruce oil combined with atlas cedar oil and peppermint oil results in a mixture that—when applied to the body after the morning shower—will, for several hours, substitute for morning coffee (see page 104).

Caution: Only use spruce oil externally!

Tarragon (*Artemisia dracunculus*)

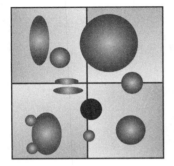

Main components: methyl chavicol
Main effects: antispasmodic
Special effects: coumarin strengthens the
antispasmodic effect
Contraindications: none when used with
caution

Tarragon oil, like exotic basil, contains estragol as well as various coumarins with names such as aesculetin, herniarin, scoparon, and scopoletin.

Like basil, it is an effective antiviral agent, but its greatest area of efficacy is as a spasmolytic. Used internally or externally, tarragon is one of aromatherapy's strongest antispasmodics.

Tea Tree (*Melaleuca alternifolia*)

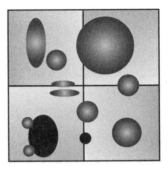

Main components: terpene alcohols
(terpinen-4-ol)
Main effects: anti-infective agent with very
broad spectrum of action
Contraindications: none known

The Australian wonder, this oil is renowned for its unbelievable antimicrobial qualities. Its wide spectrum of action makes it perfect for the traveler's first-aid kit. It is the oil perfect for treating infections of the mucous membranes of mouth and gums, for acne and herpes, and for bacterial, candida-related, or viral intestinal infections. Tea tree oil is also effective for infections of the genital area, especially chronic candida-related vaginitis, as well as infections with trichomonads.

Thyme *(Thymus vulgaris)*

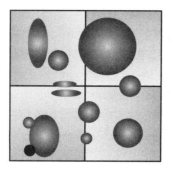

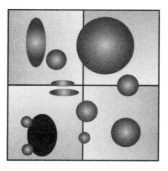

a) thyme—thymol type
Main components: phenol (thymol, carvacrol, up to 60%)
Main effects: strong anti-infective agent, stimulating, skin irritant
Contraindications: not to be used on the skin (dermocaustic)

This oil is often distilled, in whole or in part, from another plant, *Thymus zygis.* Genuine *Thymus vulgaris* is not as readily available as one might think. Through its natural content of thymol and carvacrol, *Thymus vulgaris* oil has an extremely broad spectrum of action against infectious illnesses. In its genuine state, it has a significantly more pleasant scent than most oils with an upward-adjusted phenol content.

Note: This oil should not be applied externally.

b) thyme—thujanol type
Main components: terpene alcohols (50%, thujanol and a variety of others)
Main effects: stimulating, tonic, antiviral, mild, nonirritating
Noteworthy: thujanol stimulates the liver
Contraindications: none with physiological dosages

This oil contains up to 50 percent terpene alcohols. It is one of the few oils effective against chlamydia. It is also effective against viruses and stimulates immune response as well as the regeneration of liver cells. Its broad spectrum of action against many infectious conditions makes it appropriate for a traveler's first-aid kit. Especially suitable for treating flu, bronchitis, vaginitis, cervicitis, and a general weakened condition (see pages 106, 108).

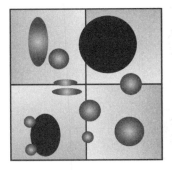

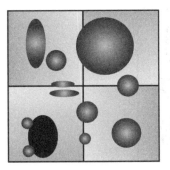

c) thyme—linalol type
Main components: terpene alcohols (linalol, 60%), esters (linalyl acetate, 20%)
Main effects: strong antiseptic, but mild on the skin
Contraindications: none with physiological dosage

In this oil the mildness of linalol and linalyl acetate is combined with the strong antiseptic action of thyme. It is excellent for impurities of the skin.

Its gentleness and antimicrobial effects have made it an aromatherapy classic overnight. It is effective against *Candida albicans* and *Staphylococcus* (stomach, intestine, cystitis), is a pleasant tonic for nervous exhaustion, and is irreplaceable in skin care.

d) thyme—geraniol type
Main components: terpene alcohols (geraniol)
Main effects: antiviral
Contraindications: none with physiological dosage

A luxury oil: very mild in its application, yet it is extremely strong and has broad action against bacteria, viruses, and fungi (yeast infections). This oil is especially suitable for use in bronchitis and viral intestinal infections. It aids falling asleep.

Vetiver (*Vetiveria zizanoides*)

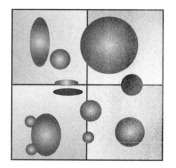

Main components: sesquiterpene-hydrocarbons, -alcohols, -ketones, esters
Main effects: tonic for arteries and veins, strengthens circulation, strengthens a weakened immune system
Contraindications: none known

This oil is often used as a fixative. Because of its active sesquiterpene-alcohols and -ketones it provides sustained stimulation for endocrine glands and circulatory system. Aromamedicine recommends vetiver for a weakened immune system.

Yarrow (*Achillea millefolium*)

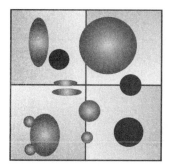

Main components: terpene hydrocarbons, chamazulene, ketones
Main effects: anti-inflammatory, cell regenerating, analgesic
Contraindications: contains ketone; *not to be used* by children less than 10 years old or pregnant women

Yarrow oils are often of deep blue color, because of a high chamazulene content. Interestingly, this is not always the case—it also often has a light yellow or green color. Yarrow oil is applied externally for neuralgia or tendinitis.

Ylang Ylang *(Cananga odorata)*

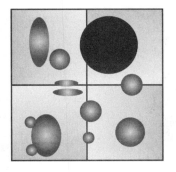

Main components: sesquiterpenes, esters ("ylang ylang extra" has a relatively higher terpene alcohol content)
Main effects: relaxing
Contraindications: none with physiological dosage

Ylang ylang oil's narcotic scent is its dominant characteristic. It is used for heart palpitations, for which even the smallest amounts, applied topically, have a remarkable effect.

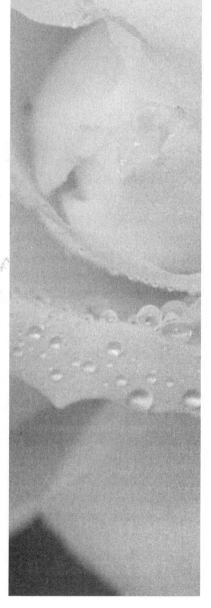

CHAPTER 6

APPLICATION OF ESSENTIAL OILS

Methods of Application

Oral Application

When taken orally, the greater part of essential oils is absorbed by the mouth or throat, the esophagus, the stomach, or the duodenum and the small intestine as the oils travel along the digestive path. From there, essential oils travel to the liver, where they are metabolized, meaning they are chemically linked to other molecules. They are thereby transformed into a water-soluble state to be processed and eliminated by the metabolism. This means their lipophilic qualities are lost, and effects tied to the lipophilic character of oils are no longer present. Research and experience have shown, however, that ingested oils still have very potent effects in the urogenital tract. Therefore, taking essential oils orally makes the most sense when we want them to interact with the liver or kidneys.

Conventional medicine typically administers medication in tablet form. But essential oil molecules, which are very small and highly lipophilic, penetrate tissue more readily, independent of how the oil is applied. Using essential oils by rubbing them into the skin or via inhalation is in many cases much more effective than oral delivery.

Essential oils can be taken in gelatin capsules or, more conveniently, taken with honey or sugar. Especially useful are peppermint and thyme (thujanol) oils because of their liver-supporting qualities—and tea tree oil—because of its antiseptic nature.

Aromatic hydrosols are often very similar in composition to their parent essential oils. They represent a naturally available hydrophilic form closest to the composition of the respective essential oil. Because of the absence of irritating qualities, they are often much better suited for ingestion than oil. One gram magnesium sulfate is dissolved in 100 milliliters hydrosol. One teaspoon of this mixture is added to a glass of water, and taken three to four times daily.

External Application

Essential oils have excellent diffusive capabilities. Rubbing or massaging an essential oil directly into the skin over an organ or area in need of treatment will provide a very high concentration of oil in the desired location. Because oils have the ability to penetrate tissue very quickly and enter the capillaries, this ensures distribution throughout the body.

An especially effective form of essential oil application is to massage the oil into the soles of the feet. With this application, immediate absorption into the the liver, as is the case when oils are ingested, is prevented, and therefore the immediate processing (linking to other molecules, making oil molecules hydrophilic) in the liver is also avoided. In this fashion essential oils reach the lower bronchial capillaries and—via the heart–lung-circulatory system—the whole or-

---

PERMEABILITY OF BODY REGIONS

Relatively permeable
Forehead
Injured or inflamed skin
Mucous membranes
Palms
Scalp
Shoulders
Soles of the feet

Relatively impermeable
Abdomen
Back
Buttocks
Chest
Legs

---

ganism unprocessed, in their original state.

Because thyme and oregano oils cannot be used in the regular topical mode, massaging these oils into the soles of the feet is especially useful for small children. Applied via the feet, thyme and oregano oils turn out to be well tolerated and highly effective.

Suppositories

The use of suppositories is well established in French aromamedicine. When oils penetrate the tissue around the rectum, they are absorbed in veins, bypassing the liver, and are consequently fed into the heart–lung-circulatory system, and from there into the circulatory system.

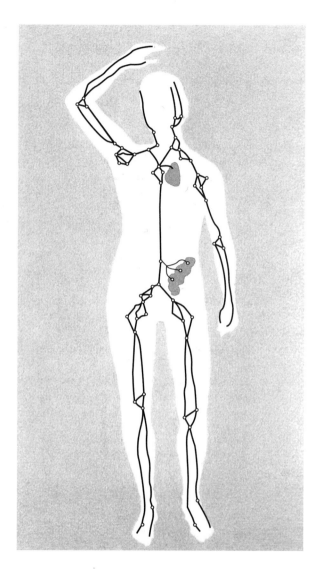

The human lymphatic system serves as a mechanism for transporting excess fluids, proteins, fats (from the intestines), and large hormone molecules. Immune cells are produced in the numerous lymph nodes.

Mouth and Throat

For disinfecting the mouth and throat essential oils can be taken in small doses (1 to 3 drops) on a charcoal tablet which is allowed to disintegrate slowly in the mouth.

For a mouthwash essential oils are mixed with a liquid food-emulsifier. A few drops in a glass of water will suffice. Dosages can be chosen according to individual tolerance and taste. Peppermint, sage, anise, and thyme are especially suited for this use.

The Nose

Hazelnut is a good carrier oil for using essential oils as nose drops. The ratio of essential oil to carrier should be about 100 milligrams per 10 milliliters base oil, which corresponds to 4 drops of essential oil in approximately 10 milliliters hazelnut oil. An especially effective method is to put a few drops of essential oil on a small square of paper towel, roll up the towel, and place it in the nostrils. Not only will the nasal passages open up, but signs of a cold will disappear overnight.

Inhalation

Electrical diffusors are suitable for inhaling essential oils. One session normally lasts between 10 and 15 minutes. For respiratory conditions it is often very effective to leave the diffusor on overnight in the bedroom at the lowest setting.

Not as involved, but very effective, is placing one drop of oil on a bed pillow, or putting some drops of oil either on a piece of paper towel and placing it directly in the nose or in an asthma inhaler and breathing through it several times a day.

Shower

One of the quickest and most effective means of application is simply to rub a small amount of es-

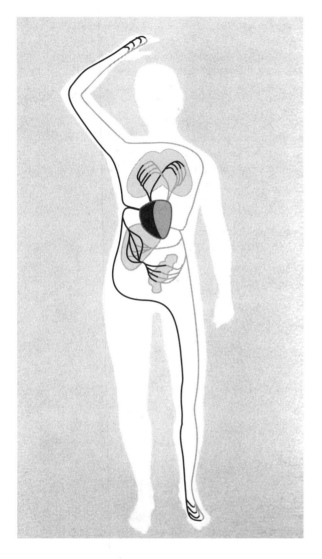

The human heart pumps oxygen-rich blood (light areas) from the lungs into the general circulatory system and oxygen-free blood (dark areas) into the heart–lung-circulatory system.

sential oil over the entire body. This is difficult when the skin is dry, as the oil is absorbed too quickly and sticks to those spots where it is first applied. To ensure a more even distribution, apply a small amount of oil (1 to 2 milliliters) while taking a shower. Do this by beginning to shower, then interrupt your shower for a moment, and apply a small amount of oil while the skin is still wet. Because of their lipophilic quality, essential oils will be absorbed instantaneously; the shower can be continued within 15 to 20 seconds.

Areas of Use

Most people who newly discover aromatherapy enter a kind of aroma-euphoria. In this euphoric state, the novice tends to try to heal all health problems—and then some—with the help of aromatherapy. Naturally, such expectations cannot be fulfilled entirely.

Aromatherapy is best suited for treating infectious illnesses. If we take into account how quickly essential oils are both absorbed by and eliminated from the body, it is not suprising that aromatherapy is most effective when quick intervention is needed, as is the case with infectious illnesses.

Aromatherapy is also effective in the areas of the psyche, nervous system, and hormonal balance. We need only think of the uplifting effects of many flower aromas, stress relief with lavender and ylang ylang, or the hormone-like effects of clary sage and geranium.

Aromatherapy is less specific in the areas of inflammatory, allergic, or autoimmune conditions, as these often develop over years or as a result of hereditary factors. Successes in these areas are likely to go along with some less dramatic results. Aromatherapy is even less effective in treating metabolic or degenerative conditions which have evolved over years and are only slowly reversible, if at all.

AUXILIARY MATERIALS

Generally there is a large degree of flexibility for combining essential oils and base materials allowing for personal preference when creating compositions and products with essential oils.

Base oils:

Almond oil is well suited for making massage or body oils. It is absorbed relatively quickly and is available at a reasonable price. Hazelnut oil is absorbed even more quickly by the skin and is a fine choice for cosmetic products. Other oils, such as avocado or sunflower oil, can also be used without problems. In general, one should choose oils that have been refined either not at all or as little as possible. Grapeseed oil, for example, is solvent extracted and therefore less suitable than cold-pressed, fatty oils.

Other base materials:

Essential oils can also be mixed with other base materials. If the fatty character of oils is to be avoided, gels are an attractive alternative. Essential oils can be added to creams or lotions either of your own manufacture or from the store. Adding oils to any existing lotion or cream slightly changes the composition of an emulsion and can lead to some separation, which generally is not a problem. Because of the skin's high permeability to essential oil components, there is a possibility that essential oils which have been mixed into

a commercial product will act as a carrier for undesirable components of the commercial products, such as polyethylene glycols (PEGs), and that such substances will enter the skin, piggybacking on the essential oils.

Charcoal tablets:

Normal charcoal tablets, available in pharmacies, are most appropriate.

Suppositories:

Cocoa butter combined with another fatty oil (such as almond or hazelnut) serves as base material for suppositories. To make suppositories, 20 grams of cocoa butter should be heated with a fatty oil (10 milliliters) in a double boiler until the cocoa butter has melted and a homogeneous mixture is formed. While this mixture is cooling, but before it has solidified, the desired essential oil (3 milliliters) is mixed in. This should be allowed to harden, then divided into appropriate portions, and each tightly wrapped in aluminum foil and stored in the freezer. Altogether, the process should take no more than 10 minutes.

Gelatin capsules:

Gelatin capsules can be filled with essential oils but are not meant to be stored that way. Freshly filled, however, they allow an aggressive or intense-tasting oil to be taken more comfortably.

SUCCESS POTENTIAL WITH AROMATHERAPY FOR:

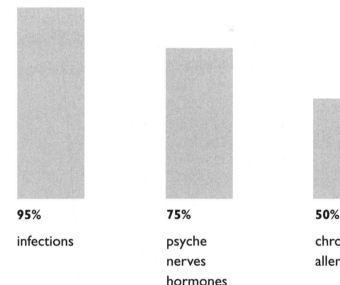

95%
infections

75%
psyche
nerves
hormones

50%
chronic inflammation
allergies

25%
metabolic conditions

Still, the possibilities for using essential oils are many and varied. The following section describes the areas most suitable for use and the possibilities for treatment with aromatherapy.

Bruises, Sprains, Sports Injuries

Everlasting oil (*Helichrysum italicum* var. *serotinum*) is certainly one of the most astounding essential oils. Its very unique chemical composition along with the essential oil's general ability to penetrate into tissue and the circulatory system permit some spectacular treatments. Used for bruises, sprains, and twisted ankles—usually accompanied by swelling and subsequent hemorrhages—this oil proves to be practically a wonder cure.

Immediately applying everlasting oil to a sprained or torn area will prevent severe swelling and bruising (hematomas).

Everlasting oil's ability to prevent swelling and bruising can be increased by mixing it with a comfrey cream or salve preparation. This oil does not just minimize swelling and bruising, but—applied directly to the injury either in pure form or diluted with a base oil—it takes away the acute pain.

Burns

For typical household or kitchen burns, generously apply lavender to the affected area and cool with ice cubes. The next day, the skin will look as if nothing had happened. With the application of lavender oil, loss of skin and a long, painful healing process can be avoided in many cases. Just as good, or perhaps even better, for this use is the oil from the bisabolol type of German chamomile.

Wounds and Scars

Everlasting oil is suitable for wound healing and for scars, resulting from either accidents or cosmetic surgery. It is especially effective when used together with rose hip seed oil. The triple unsaturated fatty acids strengthen the cell membranes and, combined with the regenerative qualities of everlasting oil, heal wounds with minimal or no scarring.

A preparation for external use:

Everlasting	0.5 milliliter
Rose hip seed oil	15 milliliters
Hazelnut oil	15 milliliters

In the French aroma literature, this combination is also recommended for slow-healing wounds and keloids as well as old, unsightly scars.

A preparation for treating old scars:

Everlasting oil	0.5 milliliter
Sage oil	0.5 milliliter
Rose hip seed oil	15 milliliters
Hazelnut oil	85 milliliters

Small, recent wounds treated two times per day for about 10 days will heal without complications. For treatment of old, unsightly scars, application is recommended over a period of 3 to 6 months.

Lymphatic System

Bay laurel oil has astounding effects on swollen lymph nodes. Experience has shown it to be very effective in supporting the lymphatic system. For various uses, see pages 74–75.

Herpes

Essential oils with a high citral or linalol content are especially effective against herpes outbreaks. Simple, topical application of 1 drop of may chang (*Litsea cubeba*) oil or especially tea tree oil will dry up blisters and reduce the recurrence of outbreaks. Fever blisters in the mouth respond well to creeping hyssop (*Hyssopus officinalis* var. *decumbens*). It is not necessary to use an expensive oil, such as melissa; equally effective is a mixture of geranium oil, *Eucalyptus radiata*, and *E. citriodora*. It is important to apply the oils undiluted to the affected area. If, after several applications within 24 to 36 hours, the skin begins to dry out and tighten, it is advisable to switch to a mixture of a fatty oil (such as hazelnut or almond) with 10 percent essential oil.

The following very effective mixture can be applied directly to the affected area three times a day:

1 part geranium oil
1 part melissa (or may chang) oil
1 part lavender oil
10 parts tea tree oil

Shingles

When it comes to treating shingles, aromatherapy has no competition. Applying a mixture of equal parts ravensare and calophyllum directly to the affected area several times a day will heal it fast and painlessly. As with herpes, shingles should be treated with aromatherapeutic measures as soon as the characteristic pain occurs prior to the outbreak of lesions. If the mixture is applied at the first sign of shingles, an outbreak can be avoided entirely or, at the very least, a significant worsening of symptoms can be lessened.

Decisively repeated treatments using essential oils will cause relapses to appear less frequently and ultimately to disappear entirely.

Bladder Infections

Tea tree is the oil of choice for treating bladder infections accompanied by a sensation of pain upon urinating. One to 3 drops of tea tree oil should be taken every half hour with lots of water or herbal tea. A significant improvement will be noticed within a few hours, and the pain should be gone within 1 to 3 days. But, although tea tree oil has such good results, one should try to identify the true causes of the infection in order to avoid them in the future. If symptoms persist, a physician should be consulted.

Bloodshot Eyes and Conjunctivitis

The watery environment of the eyes and the very sensitive nature of the mucous membranes prohibit the use of essential oils in the eye area. However, the aromatic hydrosol of green myrtle is perfectly suited for any inflammation of the eyes. It is easy to use: with the eyes closed, one should spray small amounts of myrtle water on closed eyelids. Inexperienced users will blink while spraying; "professionals" will spray directly into the open eye.

Nervousness, Tension, Stress

Nervousness, tension, and stress call for the sedative qualities of aldehydes, the diverse action of ester components on the central nervous system, and the sympatholytic effects (calming, dilation of blood vessels, lowering blood pressure) of some phenylpropanes. Stress dissipates.

For cramps and tense muscles (topical):

Tarragon	I milliliter
Cypress	I milliliter
Thyme, thujanol type	I milliliter
Marjoram	2 milliliters
Gel or oil base	50 milliliters

Use 1 to 2 milliliters of this mixture with each application up to 5 times per day.

For stress and anxiety:

Mandarin	I milliliter
Mandarin petitgrain	I milliliter
Lemon verbena	I milliliter

Rub 1 or 2 drops of this mixture on the temples and above the solar plexus. This mixture can be used repeatedly as often as necessary.

For nervous tension:

Marjoram	I milliliter
Ylang ylang	I milliliter
Mandarin	I milliliter

Take 1 to 3 drops of this mixture in a capsule (see page 100) several times daily.

These recipes should serve only as general guidelines. The oils can be combined according to individual needs and tastes. Listed below are some of the most important oils and their uses in the area of stress.

- Spasmolytic: tarragon, Roman chamomile, ylang ylang

- Sedative: lemon verbena, melissa, spikenard, mandarin petitgrain
- Balancing: lavender, clary sage

Finally, a recipe for anyone who is under extreme stress.

For extreme stress:

Roman chamomile	1 milliliter
Clary sage	1 milliliter
Mandarin petitgrain	1 milliliter
Spikenard	1 milliliter
Hazelnut oil	10 milliliters

Apply this combination to the wrists, elbows, and temples and above the solar plexus. One application should be enough to achieve the desired effects, but repeated use is not hazardous.

Motion Sickness

One drop of peppermint oil is the ideal remedy for nauseated children in the back seat of a car traveling over curvy mountain passes. Most adults and youngsters over twelve can handle 1 drop of pure oil, but children under twelve should take peppermint diluted, for example, on a piece of sugar. The effect will last longer if the air in the car has been scented with a few drops of peppermint oil. Conventional medicine has confirmed the effectiveness of peppermint against irritable colon.

Fatigue

For those individuals who believe they need copious amounts of coffee to get through the fast-paced, heartless workday, aromatherapy offers sensible, holistic help: For this, one should mix equal parts *Pinus sylvestris* and *Picea mariana* and add this combination to a base oil so that the essential oils comprise 10 percent of the final mixture. This mixture is applied on the area over the kidneys. These oils strengthen the functions of the adrenal glands, without overstimulating them the way coffee does. This mixture can also be expanded to provide a stimulating morning lotion by mixing the two needle oils with some Atlas cedar and citrus oils according to individual preference. A 5 percent solution in a body lotion can be applied all over the body after the morning shower. This will make coffee's stimulating effects obsolete.

For adrenal support:

Black spruce	5 milliliters
Atlas cedar	2 milliliters
Peppermint oil	1 milliliter
Hazelnut oil (or lotion)	100 milliliters

Infectious Illnesses

Dr. Jean Valnet held the opinion that the role of microorganisms in infectious illnesses is greatly overestimated. In the language of his day, this meant that the condition of the "terrain" in which the microorganism tries to spread is equally as important as the process of the infection itself. We can see this, for example, when several people exposed to the same bacteria become ill, while others do not.

In French aromamedicine, as well as in other areas of alternative medicine, it is accepted that acute and chronic illnesses originate in imbalances of the intestinal flora. "Beneficial" bacteria ensure a healthy balance; without them, infections of all kinds would run rampant. There are also beneficial bacteria present in the mouth, on the skin, in the vagina, and in the intestines. The good bacteria on the skin secrete substances which protect the body from bacterial and fungal infections. *Lactobacillus* bacteria, in the small intestine and vagina, protect the body from yeast and bacterial invasions. One of the problems with antibiotics is that they indiscriminately kill beneficial and pathogenic bacteria, leaving the body unprotected.

The digestive tract is host to countless species of microorganisms which, in ideal circumstances, coexist in a harmonious symbiosis. These organisms carry out many important functions for our health. Bacteria such as *Lactobacillus acidophilus* or *Bifidobacterium bifidus* help digestion, synthesize vitamins, and defend against pathogenic bacteria. Beneficial bacteria help prevent infection and, just by their presence on the intestinal wall, take up space that would otherwise be inhabited by pathogenic germs. If no good bacteria were present, pathogenic germs would reproduce unchecked.

If the sensitive balance of intestinal flora is disrupted by pathogenic germs for example, liver and kidneys are placed under increased stress. Toxins from the metabolism of the pathogens, but also from food and environment, overburden the eliminating organs. They are no longer able to eliminate the flood of toxins through normal means. Excess toxins are stored in various parts of the body, effectively creating toxic waste deposits. Finally, under the increasing pressure of a continually increasing toxic load, they are transported to "emergency elimination sites," for instance to the skin or to the mucous membranes. The elimination of toxins through the skin, through mucous membranes, through the sinus cavities or bronchi creates the breeding ground (mucus, pus) for secondary bacterial infections and the corresponding inflammations. This is a simplified outline, but it does describe the essence of the situation. In the words of Daniel Pénoël: "All illnesses which end in the suffix *itis*, such as bronchitis, are emergency reactions of the body to eliminate excess toxins."

Based on this understanding, French aromamedicine since Belaiche's time has developed a method that aims first to cleanse the inflamed area with mucolytic oils from elimination products (mucus, pus) to prevent the onset of secondary bacterial infections and to initiate the reestablishment of healthy conditions. In a second step, a combination of antiseptic essences prohibits the spread of viruses and bacteria acting against the remaining pathogens.

Principles of phytomedical infection treatment

The three-step phytotherapeutic (Greek *phyto*, meaning plant) treatment of bacterial and fungal infections, especially those characterized by the buildup of mucus or pus, is as follows:

1. Treatment from day 1 to day 3

If germs reproduce on catarrhal excretions, such as pus or mucus, the affected areas must first be cleansed and disinfected with mucolytic oils and/or hydrosols.

2. Antiseptic treatment, from day 4 to day 7

In the second phase, any remaining pathogenic germs are eliminated with alternating applications of mucolytic, microbicidal, or fungicidal essential oils or hydrosols. This method is especially effective since many of the mucolytic essential oils, such as rosemary (verbenone type) or *Inula graveolens*, also have a distinct antimicrobial effect. Phases 1 and 2 use essential oils which stimulate the elimination of mucus and pus.

Essences used for topical disinfection may also be taken internally if necessary in more serious cases. To support the lymphatic system, Cistus (*Cistus ladaniferus*) and Laurel (*Laurus nobilis*) can be applied on the lymph nodes, in addition to the measures given above.

3. Postacute strengthening treatment— convalescence, from day 8 to day 28

After the acute symptoms of the infectious illness have clearly improved (normally, after about 1 week), small amounts of essential oils supporting convalescence are used. Essential oils that have been shown effective in an aromatogram for a particular patient should also be used. In an aromamedical treatment, the doctor or patient will choose those oils which improve immune status, support liver function, and restore hormonal balance.

The self-medicating aromatherapy user working without the help of an aromatogram can fall back on oils that are principally suitable for supporting the liver function in convalescence. These are oils with a high concentration of terpene alcohols, sesquiterpenes, and sesquiterpene alcohols: thyme (thujanol type), carrot seed, and Greenland moss.

An application suggested by Franchomme and Pénoël consists of taking 50 milligrams (about 2 drops) of carrot seed oil and/or 50 milligrams thyme (thujanol type) in a gelatin capsule at lunchtime, and 50 milligrams Greenland moss

oil in the evening. These oils should always be taken either with meals or in gelatin-capsule form over a period of 3 weeks.

The table on page 107 gives a systematic overview of this method of treatment. It shows the effective essential oil components and the essential oils typically used in each phase of the treatment.

Respiratory Conditions (air passages, throat, nose, ears)

The following recommendations for treatment are contributions of Dr. Pénoël to the *Aromatherapy Course* of the Pacific Institute of Aromatherapy.

Bronchitis with secondary bacterial infection and catarrh (severe bronchitis accompanied by mucus)

Phase 1: mucolytic treatment

Rosemary, verbenone type	1.5 milliliters
Eucalyptus dives	.75 milliliter
Suppository base	30 milliliters (sufficient for 10 suppositories)

Two suppositories per day. These dosages are good for adults. Use the same mixture for children, but use only suppositories half or a third the size, depending on the child's age.

For mucolytic inhalation rosemary (verbenone type) is inhaled for 5 minutes every hour in aerosol form (from a diffusor). The oil is also rubbed onto the upper body. Combining these applications is the best way to utilize the mucolytic and antibacterial properties of this oil.

GENERAL TREATMENT PRINCIPLES FOR INFECTIOUS ILLNESSES

Days 1 to 3: Phase 1

Using oils with mucolytic and expectorant qualities to cleanse the mucous membranes.

MUCOLYTIC COMPONENTS
Ketones in:
Eucalyptus dives
Rosemary, verbenone type

Lactones in:
Inula graveolens

EXPECTORANTS
Cineole in:
Myrtle
Ravensare aromatica
Laurel
Eucalyptus globulus
Eucalyptus radiata

Days 4 to 7: Phase 2

Eliminating remaining pathogens with oils with bactericidal and fungicidal components.
Phases 1 and 2 can be alternated during the first 7 days of treatment.

BACTERICIDAL COMPONENTS
Monoterpene alcohols in:
Ravensare aromatica
Niaouli
Tea tree
Eucalyptus radiata

Phenols in:
Mountain savory
Thyme
Oregano

FUNGICIDAL COMPONENTS
Esters in:
Lavender
Roman chamomile
Geranium

Days 8 to 21: Phase 3

Supporting convalescence. Essences with a sesquiterpene-alcohol and -ketone content
are especially suited for this phase.

LIVER-STIMULATING
Sesquiterpene alcohols in:
Carrot seed oil
Greenland moss

IMMUNE-REGULATING
Melissa (for infections)
Lemon (for drainage)
Tarragon (for cramps)

Phase 2: infection treatment

Thyme, thymol type	1.25 milliliters
Oregano	1.25 milliliters
Suppository base	30 milliliters
	(sufficient for 10
	suppositories)

Two suppositories per day. Amounts given are for adults. Use the same mixture for children, but use only suppositories half or a third the size, depending on the child's age.

A mild, but effective complement to the suppository mixture is a blend of mild antiseptic oils, which are rubbed into the skin.

Thyme, thujanol type	4 milliliters
Myrtle, cineole type	2 milliliters

Apply 10 to 15 drops of this mixture several times daily.

Phase 3: supporting convalescence

Thyme, thujanol type	
(or carrot seed)	1 drop

To be taken at lunchtime. If available, 1 drop of Greenland moss is taken in the evening with syrup or in a capsule, according to taste.

Viral bronchitis

For bronchitis without a secondary infection (coughing without significant mucus, with mild or no fever), it is often sufficient to ease the progression with antiviral oils. This will usually prevent worsening due to secondary infection. The following suppository treatment is well suited.

Creeping hyssop	1.5 milliliters

Thyme, linalol type	0.5 milliliter
Suppository base	30 milliliters
	(sufficient for 10
	suppositories)

Up to 8 suppositories per day in acute cases. This mixture is mild enough to be used for small children. Creeping hyssop is especially useful for its mucolytic and spasmolytic effects in the lower bronchial area.

Dilation of the bronchi and capillaries (emphysema)

If, in addition to infectious bronchitis, emphysema is present, topical application of pine and cypress oils is useful.

Pine	6 milliliters
Cypress	4 milliliters
Hazelnut oil	10 milliliters
Gel, or oil base	100 milliliters

Rub onto chest two or three times per day.

Catarrh (cold in the nose and throat with secondary bacterial infection and excess mucus)

Phase 1:

Rosemary, verbenone type	5 milliliters
Eucalyptus globulus	2 milliliters
Peppermint	3 drops
	(sufficient for
	about 15 doses)

Inhale several times a day, in the form of diffusor aerosol or directly off a cloth. Because of its ketone content, rosemary (verbenone type) is generally used as a mucolytic with minimal toxicity.

Phase 2:

Thyme, linalol type	9 milliliters
Creeping hyssop	2 milliliters

For inhalation or to be massaged into the skin.

Phase 3:

Thyme, thujanol type (or carrot seed)	1 drop

To be taken with lunch. If available, 1 drop of Greenland moss is taken in the evening with syrup or in a capsule.

Colds (viral rhinitis and rhinopharyngitis)

Light catarrhal conditions without secondary infection, or sniffles marking the beginning of a cold, respond to antiviral oils used to prevent the condition from developing into a full-blown cold or bronchitis. The following mixtures are used parallel and/or alternately:

Eucalyptus radiata	5 milliliters
Eucalyptus globulus	2.5 milliliters
Ravensare	2.5 milliliters

This mixture is best inhaled with a diffusor, for 5 to 10 minutes six times daily. If no diffusor is available, 5 drops should be placed on a cloth and inhaled directly, several times an hour in acute cases.

Eucalyptus radiata	2 milliliters
Eucalyptus globulus	1 milliliter
Calophyllum	5 milliliters
Gel or oil base	100 milliliters

This mixture is used as nose drops. Through inhalation and local topical application, a cold is treated effectively without taking oils internally.

Peppermint	2 milliliters
Tea tree	1 milliliter
Thyme, linalol type	1 milliliter

Put some drops of this oil mixture onto a piece of paper towel, roll, and put into the nostril(s) before bedtime.

Sinus infection

The phase 1 mucolytic treatment, for 2 to 4 days, is done with *Inula graveolens* and peppermint. If *Inula* is not available, rosemary (verbenone type) is used.

Phase 1:

Inula graveolens or rosemary, verbenone type	1 milliliter
Peppermint	1 drop

To be inhaled several times daily.

Phase 2:

Anti-infective treatment over 3 to 4 days by inhalation and internal use of essential oils.

Mixture 1: inhalation	
Eucalyptus radiata	5 milliliters
Spike lavender	1 milliliter (sufficient for 7 sessions)

Mixture 2: to be taken orally	
Thyme, thujanol type	3 milliliters
Thyme, thymol type	3 drops

A carbon tablet or similar carrier with 1 to 3 drops of the mixture is allowed to disintegrate slowly in the mouth. This is done up to six times daily.

Phase 3:

Days 4 to 7. External application of decongesting oils reducing mucus secretion.

Pine	I milliliter
Cypress	0.5 milliliter
Hazelnut oil, or gel	3 milliliters

The oil should be massaged over the sinuses.

Whooping cough

Phase 1:

The following applications are carried out simultaneously:

Mixture I: to be taken orally

Marjoram	I milliliter
Syrup, or similar	100 milliliters

One drop to be taken every half hour.

Mixture 2: to be applied topically

Cypress	5 milliliters
Hazelnut oil	5 milliliters
Base oil	50 milliliters

To be massaged over the upper body every half hour.

Phase 2:

Marjoram	I.5 milliliters
Thyme, thujanol type	I.5 milliliters
Suppository mixture	30 milliliters

These suppositories can be given every half hour, but at least every 3 hours, until symptoms improve. Maximum of 10 suppositories per day.

Phase 3:

Thyme, thujanol type (or carrot seed oil)	I drop

To be taken at lunchtime. If available, 1 drop of Greenland moss oil is taken in the evening with syrup or in a capsule, according to taste.

Middle ear infection

Phase 1 and phase 2 can be carried out simultaneously.

Phase 1:

Inula graveolens or rosemary, verbenone type	I milliliter
Peppermint	I drop

This mixture is massaged around the ear, along the lymph nodes, and onto the neck.

Phase 2:

Eucalyptus radiata	8 milliliters
Spike lavender	2 milliliters

This mixture can be sprayed as an aerosol into the ear, or 2 drops can be put on a cotton ball, and left in the ear for a minute or two.

If the condition and pain persist and there is no improvement after 48 hours, the treatment should be intensified with 1 to 3 suppositories of the following mixture:

Thyme, thymol type	I milliliter
Mountain savory	I milliliter
Suppository base	20 milliliters (sufficient for I0 suppositories)

This quantity is good for adult suppositories. For children, use the following total amounts of oil mixture (instead of the combination shown above): for children between 6 and 12, use $^1/_2$ milliliter; for children over 12 years, use $1^1/_2$ milliliters.

Phase 3:

Thyme, thymol type (or carrot seed)	I drop

To be taken at lunchtime. If available, 1 drop of Greenland moss is taken in the evening, with syrup or sorbet, or in a capsule, according to taste.

Tonsillitis

For serious infections a mixture of essential oils with high phenol concentrations should be used.

Phase 1:

Mountain savory	I milliliter
Thyme, thymol type	I milliliter
Clove	5 drops

A charcoal tablet with 2 drops of the mixture is allowed to disintegrate slowly in the mouth, three to four times a day. If this mixture of phenolic oils proves too strong or irritating, use the following aromatic water.

Hydrosol:

Mountain savory water (aromatic hydrosol of *Satureja montana*)	50 milliliters
Thyme water (aromatic hydrosol of *Thymus vulgaris*, thymol type)	40 milliliters

Spray this hydrosol mixture in the mouth every 15 to 30 minutes for several hours.

Phase 2:

A milder mixture for less serious infections.

Thyme, linalol type	I milliliter
Thyme, thujanol type	I milliliter

A charcoal tablet with 2 drops of the mixture is allowed to disintegrate slowly in the mouth, three to four times a day.

Phase 3:

Thyme, thujanol type (or carrot seed)	I drop

To be taken at lunchtime. If available, 1 drop of Greenland moss oil is taken in the evening with syrup or in a capsule, according to taste.

Convulsive cough (croup)

It is crucial to quell the coughing impulse with the following mixtures, to be taken simultaneously:

Mixture I:

Tarragon	I milliliter
Syrup	100 milliliters

One teaspoon to be taken every 15 to 30 minutes.

Mixture 2:

Dill	5 milliliters
Hazelnut oil	5 milliliters
Gel or oil base	40 milliliters

To be rubbed into the chest as often as coughing attacks require.

Hay fever

Hay fever is an allergic condition of the respiratory tract which can be effectively ameliorated with the following oil mixtures. Using these mixtures in a diffusor requires caution because they can provoke strong reactions. In the context of allergic conditions it is wise to consider using aromatic hydrosols, which are milder and involve lower risk than essential oils, especially when the primary site of the allergy is treated.

Myrtle, cineole type	5 milliliters
Creeping hyssop	1.5 milliliters
German chamomile	3 drops (sufficient for 100 applications)

A charcoal tablet with 1 to 3 drops of this mixture is allowed to disintegrate slowly in the mouth, three to four times a day. (The charcoal tablets can be substituted with any other absorbent material which allows for a slow release of the oils in the mouth.)

Hydrosol:

Myrtle water (aromatic hydrosol of *Myrtus communis*)	80 milliliters
Cistus water (aromatic hydrosol of *Cistus ladaniferus*)	20 milliliters

It is advantageous to use this mixture as a spray, to better reach nasal and throat passages. For application in the eyes, either as a spray or in an eye wash, the mixture should be diluted with equal amounts of sterilized, distilled water.

Sterilizing water: bring distilled water to a boil, carefully pour into bottle with tight-fitting lid, and let cool.

Skin Conditions

Unless otherwise stated, in all components of the following mixtures the ratio is 1:1. If you would like to alter the scent somewhat, you may change the ratio of one oil or another, as long as the total concentration of essential oils in the base remains within 0.5 to 5 percent. In general the lowest oil concentrations are desirable as they tend to provide the strongest effects. If preferred, an oil-free synthetic gel can be substituted for fatty oils such as almond or hazelnut.

Bacterial dermatitis

Thyme, thujanol type	4 milliliters
Tea tree oil	4 milliliters
Eucalyptus globulus	4 milliliters
Gel base	60 milliliters

To be applied externally to afflicted areas three to five times daily.

Additionally:

Thyme, thujanol type	1 drop
Palmarosa	1 drop
Eucalyptus globulus	1 drop

To be taken in a teaspoon of vegetable oil, or in a capsule, three times per day for 8 to 10 days.

Skin infections with pus

Undiluted tea tree oil is applied directly to the affected areas up to five times per day.

Fungal skin infections

Tea tree oil, the standard treatment for fungal conditions, may not be effective against fungus which has worked its way under the toenails. Skillfully combining oils can increase their effects.

Thyme, thymol type	4 milliliters
Oregano	2 milliliters
Cinnamon oil	2 milliliters

Add 5 milliliters of this mixture to 15 milliliters of base oil. This mixture will most likely get rid of the most stubborn fungus if applied two times per day for up to 14 days. Application should not be continued if clear improvement is not visible after 2 weeks.

An alternative recipe:

Palmarosa	1 milliliter
Eucalyptus globulus	1 milliliter
Thyme, thujanol type	1 milliliter
Fatty base oil	100 milliliters

Two to four applications per day for a period of 10 to 14 days.

Candida-related yeast infections are effectively contained with the regimen oulined below:

One starts with high dosages of oregano, reduces it on the third and again on the fourth day, and continues treatment with essential oils with a high terpene alcohol content. The body often reacts to the oregano treatment with a typical "die-off" reaction. Elimination of the dead yeasts is accompanied by nausea and headaches. Even though treatment of candida with essential oils is extremely effective, one should always ask whether careless antibiotic use was the cause (and avoid it in the future).

Dry eczema

Lavender	1 milliliter
Palmarosa	1 milliliter
Calophyllum	10 milliliters
Rose hip seed oil	30 milliliters

Three to four applications per day directly to the affected area. This mixture relieves itchiness and stimulates regeneration of skin tissue.

Weeping eczema

Thyme, thujanol type	1 milliliter
Eucalyptus citriodora	1 milliliter
Calophyllum	10 milliliters
Rose hip seed oil	30 milliliters

Three to four topical applications per day on the affected areas.

Slow-healing wounds

Everlasting	1 milliliter
Sage	1 milliliter
Rose hip seed oil	15 milliliters
Hazelnut oil	15 milliliters

Two applications per day for 10 days on recent wounds, or for 3 to 6 months for old scars.

Varicose veins and related conditions

Laurel	1 milliliter
Calophyllum	30 milliliters
Rose hip seed oil	30 milliliters

Three applications externally per day for period of 7 to 14 days. This mixture utilizes the anti-infective qualities of laurel oil with the regenerating qualities of rose hip seed oil.

Also effective is laurel hydrosol. It is applied three to four times daily in a cold compress.

Hematoma (bruises)

Everlasting	5 milliliters
Calophyllum	1 milliliter

Four to six local applications per day. This mixture is effective for new and old bruises alike.

Cellulite

Eucalyptus citriodora	2 milliliters
Lemon	2 milliliters
Cedarwood	2 milliliters
Sage	2 milliliters
Cypress	2 milliliters
Niaouli (MQV)	2 milliliters
Hazelnut oil	100 milliliters

Two to three external applications daily for a period of 30 days. This mixture stimulates circulation.

Preventing stretch marks

Mandarin	4 milliliters
Rose hip seed oil	20 milliliters
Hazelnut oil	200 milliliters

To be massaged into the skin from the second through ninth months of pregnancy.

Healing stretch marks

Sage	1 milliliter
Rosemary, verbenone type	2 milliliters
Rose hip seed oil	20 milliliters
Hazelnut oil	40 milliliters

For healing stretch marks from a previous pregnancy. To be massaged into the skin with a loofah sponge for a period of 3 to 6 months.

Warts

Small warts often disappear with a drop of thuja oil applied locally. Other effective oils are thyme (thujanol type), clove, and oregano.

It is important to note that an apparent increase in the size of the wart often signals the beginning of the healing process. Those parts of the wart hidden beneath the skin are rejected by the healing tissue and are pushed outward.

Cosmetics with Natural Substances

The trend in medicine of placing more and more trust in plant-derived ingredients is being reflected in the cosmetics industry as well. This stems from discoveries regarding the biological and physiological properties of medicinal plants.

Plants offer an easily accessible source for highly active components best suited for the human organism. In contrast to the effects of synthetic products, adverse side effects are rarely observed. Most of the synthetic substances used in cosmetics today do not take part in metabolic processes of cell reproduction, and cause undesired or toxic effects if used over a significant period. In contrast, plant-derived products are active and have remarkable therapeutic effects if used with the proper cosmetic base material.

It is concurrent with the holistic viewpoint to consider the appearance of the skin, nails, hair, and eyelashes as indicators of the body's and metabolism's general state of well-being. A healthy appearance depends on a properly functioning digestive tract and a good balance in the circulatory and nervous systems, all of which in turn depend on a healthy hormonal balance. A successful cosmetic treatment depends on a healthy metabolism and good eating habits.

Essential oils, aromatic waters, and other natural substances are well suited for skin care, but a realistic outlook must be maintained toward the regeneration and rejuvenation of skin.

It is possible though to have a positive influence on stress-related skin problems in a relatively short period of time if genuine and authentic essential oils are used. While normal cosmetic treatment is symptom-oriented and attempts to change the skin in one way or another, the goal of essential oil treatment is always the restoration of balance. Treatment with essential oils attempts to bring the metabolic functions back into balance. It is not the purpose of holistic essential oil cosmetics to encourage the expectation of miracles as promised by the mainstream cosmetics industry.

As is so often the case, inner attitude is of the utmost importance; in aroma cosmetics we should keep in mind not just cosmetic effects but the whole person.

Classic oil mixtures for skin care

Provided below are aroma cosmetic compositions, as well as the conditions and circumstances which contributed to the success of these classic mixtures.

Below is a discussion of the conditions that aroma cosmetics must meet to be successful:

1. Effectiveness

Of the conditions necessary for successful aroma cosmetics, most important is the effectiveness of a particular mixture. In our fast-paced times, we look for preparations that produce well-being and positive results in the shortest possible time. Since 1985 the conditions for creating effective essential oil mixtures have been especially positive. Instead of insufficiently defined oils prepared for the fragrance industry, now oils perfectly tailored for use in holistic cosmetic preparations are available. In addition to basil, lemon, and clary

sage, it is now also possible to use special chemotypes of thyme and rosemary with their well-defined application spectrum. Oils with strong anti-allergenic properties, such as German chamomile, have since found their way into aromatherapeutic skin care.

2. Problem-free application

Besides effectiveness, a high degree of safety is required. This means essential oil compositions for cosmetic purposes must not cause skin irritations or allergic reactions, even in subjects predisposed to such reactions. The extremely high tolerability explains the compositions' continued success over many years.

How is this high degree of tolerability achieved? Experience has shown that, as a rule, use of correct genuine, pure essential oils does not cause negative side effects. The allergenic potential of essential oils often described in literature seems to stem from a basic misunderstanding: conventional oils manufactured for the flavor and fragrance industry show a much larger potential for causing allergic reactions than do genuine oils.

A great deal of circumstantial evidence indicates that undesired reactions caused by cosmetic aroma products are due not to the implicated molecules, such as geraniol, but to undefined and unknown impurities which find their way into essential oils when they are standardized with synthetic substances.

Safety is first and foremost assured by using oils of defined botanical origin whose producer and vendor are known. This assures that an oil has not been produced for the conventional market, but especially for aromatherapy use. In terms of French aromamedicine, safe use of the essential oils and full exploitation of the precisely characterized spectrum of their effects is only possible with the exclusive use of genuine oils.

All of the following compositions are products which consist of only hazelnut oil as a base material and the essential oils listed. These products have been on the market in the United States since 1985, and they have proven themselves to be extremely safe and tolerable.

Day and night care for normal skin

This mixture was originally conceived as a treatment for acne. Because of its effectiveness, its pleasant feel to the skin, and its intriguing aromas, it garnered such popularity that it became the standard day and night care for healthy and normal skin.

Thyme, linalol type	0.5 milliliter
Rosemary, verbenone type	0.5 milliliter
Neroli	0.5 milliliter
Spike lavender	0.5 milliliter
Hazelnut oil	50 milliliters

Thyme (linalol type; *Thymus vulgaris*) combines the strong antiseptic properties of thyme with non-irritant qualities and a more attractive scent than is found with thyme oils of high phenol content. In the interaction with the other components of this mixture, this oil controls microorganisms.

Rosemary (verbenone type; *Rosmarinus officinalis*) stimulates regeneration of skin cells. Rosemary displays its main activity in the dermis (the middle layer of skin), where it stimulates metabolic functions, circulation, and the elimination of waste products.

Neroli (*Citrus aurantium*—bitter orange flower) lends this composition a luxurious scent.

The specific effects of spike lavender (*Lavandula latifolia*) are described under the recipe for treating skin impurities.

Care for sensitive skin, chemically damaged or sunburned skin, and spider veins (broken capillaries)

This is one of the most successful rejuvenating mixtures for regenerative skin care in the tradition of French aromamedicine. What makes it so unique for sensitive skin and spider veins is that, through the interaction of regenerating and anti-inflammatory components, it creates the necessary stimulation of the skin without causing irritation. This mixture strengthens the rejuvenative capabilities of the skin. It is suitable for sunburn and any chemically caused irritation or injuries of sensitive and very sensitive skin.

Moroccan chamomile	0.5 milliliter
Everlasting	0.5 milliliter
Lavender	0.5 milliliter
Roman chamomile	0.5 milliliter
Hazelnut oil	50 milliliters

The blue color of this mixture stems from the Moroccan chamomile (*Tanacetum annuum*), which, due to its azulene content, has spectacular anti-inflammatory properties.

Everlasting (*Helichrysum italicum* var. *serotinum*) is, along with German chamomile, one of the strongest anti-inflammatory oils in aromatherapy. Moroccan chamomile and everlasting complement each other's effects, and everlasting has the added value of stimulating the formation of new cells.

Lavender (*Lavandula angustifolia*) harmonizes the composition and simultaneously relieves emotional tension through the effects of its esters on the nervous system.

If skin has been overstimulated or injured, tension or spasms often are observed as a reaction. Roman chamomile, in turn strengthened by the esters of lavender, counteracts these.

Vitalizing care for pallid skin

Dull, pallid skin, lifeless and tired from environmental stress, essentially healthy but lacking tonus, is best served by the following mixture. It is based on the regenerating, stimulating qualities of carrot seed oil.

Carrot seed oil	0.5 milliliter
Lemon verbena	0.5 milliliter
Niaouli	0.5 milliliter
Rosemary, verbenone type	0.5 milliliter
Hazelnut oil	50 milliliters

Carrot seed (*Daucus carota*) is one of the strongest revitalizing essential oils, due in part to substances which can be considered precursors of carotene.

Niaouli oil, or MQV (*Melaleuca quinquenervia viridiflora*), is one of the most versatile essential oils. Its spectrum of action includes anti-allergenic and antiseptic effects. In skin care, it is used for its firming effect on the skin tissue.

Rosemary (verbenone type; *Rosmarinus officinalis*) displays its main action primarily on the dermal layer of the skin, where it stimulates metabolism and detoxification.

The citral in lemon verbena (*Lippia citriodora*) has a decidedly stimulating effect on the skin tissue and contributes to the removal of toxins. It is interesting that genuine *Lippia citriodora*, unlike other oils with similar concentrations of citral, does not irritate the skin.

Care for overactive (oily) skin

The following mixture is intended for overactive skin and for acne caused by overactive sebaceous glands. It treats overactive skin without damaging the skin's protective hydrolipid layer, and avoids the constant removal of sebum, thereby reducing the stimulation of the skin to constantly replace the removed sebum.

Inula graveolens (or green myrtle)	0.5 milliliter
Eucalyptus dives	0.5 milliliter
Spike lavender	0.5 milliliter
Rosemary, verbenone type	0.5 milliliter
Hazelnut, base oil	50 milliliters

The heart and soul of this preparation is the emerald green *Inula graveolens*. It is valued for its mucolytic properties in treating respiratory conditions. In this application, it dissolves hardened sebum from clogged glands. (If *Inula graveolens* is not available, green myrtle can be substituted instead.)

Eucalyptus (piperitone type; *Eucalyptus dives*) is traditionally used to calm hyperactive sebaceous glands.

Camphor's stimulating effects on skin tissue are well known; nevertheless, the risks associated with it make use of pure camphor unwise. An ideal way to integrate camphor into skin care is the use of spike lavender. In its natural state this oil contains about 10 percent camphor. Embedded into a matrix of balancing and calming components, as they are known from *Lavandula vera*, the aggressiveness of camphor is ameliorated and its positive properties can be uitilized without risk.

Rosemary (verbenone type; *Rosmarinus officinalis*) lends its well-known regenerating effects to this mixture.

Care for aging skin

Cistus and green myrtle are used for existing or imminent wrinkles around the eyes. Since, after being applied to the area around the eye, essential oils can quickly migrate into the eyes and cause irritation, the concentration of the oils is very low.

Green myrtle	0.5 milliliter
Cistus	0.5 milliliter
Rose hip seed oil	20 milliliters
Hazelnut oil	200 milliliters

The oil of rock rose (*Cistus ladaniferus)* is produced in hot, sun-drenched regions. It is used in aromamedicine for its astringent and tightening qualities. Rock rose is the fastest-acting oil to stop bleeding from open wounds and, with its masculine scent, it is perfectly suited for men to close small cuts after shaving. Dr. Pénoël has used rock rose with great success to stop internal bleeding.

Green myrtle (cineole type; *Myrtus communis*) has been selected not only for its tonic properties but also to round out the mixture's scent. If intended for use in and around the eyes, the oils in this mixture should make up no more than 0.5 percent of the total combination. Further, to maintain elasticity of the skin, and generally to support the integrity of the cell membrane, it is advisable to add a fair amount (approximately 10 percent of the mixture) of oils containing triple unsaturated fatty acids. The best and most reasonably priced is rose hip seed oil.

CHAPTER 7

AROMATHERAPY: MEDIATING BETWEEN THE IMMUNE SYSTEM, EMOTIONS, AND THE BODY

Aromatherapy and the Immune System

Precise statements about the specific interaction between essential oils and the various functions of the immune system are not possible at this time. However, some promising developments have emerged in this area. It is probable that, with the increasing popularity of aromatherapy, in the near future a field known as "aroma-immunology" may arise because certain conclusions about the relationship between oils and their effects on the immune system can already be drawn. Immunoglobulin levels in the bloodstream, for example, can be positively influenced by treatment with essential oils.[1] Although studies in this area are still preliminary, and the details can only be presented in a very simplified manner, they hold enough promise for the future to be mentioned.[2] Various terpene alcohols have the ability to correct pathologically elevated or depressed gamma-globulin counts to their proper level. A depressed gamma-globulin level, as is encountered with chronic bronchitis, can be corrected upward with savory, thyme (linalol type), spike lavender, and *Eucalyptus globulus*. In the opposite case, where "immune depression" is expressed by a hyperstimulation of gamma globulins which have

OIL COMPONENT	IMMUNOGLOBULINS			COMMENT
	α-globulin	**β-globulin**	**γ-globulin**	
Phenols			increases	immune-stimulating
Aldehydes	reduces	reduces	reduces	anti-inflammatory
Estragol	increases	increases	reduces	modulating
Ketones	reduces	increases	reduces	modulating
Monoterpenes	reduces		reduces	modulating
Monoterpene alcohols			equilibrating	modulating

no positive effect on the inflammative process, oils with terpene alcohols normalize the pathologically elevated levels downward. Especially effective in the latter case is borneol, which is found abundantly in Moroccan thyme (*Thymus satureioides*).

If aromatherapy is to be used for immune insufficiency, Franchomme recommends the following approach: The treatment is initiated with 500 milligrams oregano or thyme (thymol chemotype) oil, divided into 10 applications of 50 milligrams each for the first and second day. On the third day, the dosage of the phenol-containing oil (oregano or thyme) is halved and combined with 250 milligrams of a terpene alcohol–containing oil. On the fourth day the dosage of the phenolic oils is again cut in half and the amount of terpene-alcohol oils increased respectively. From the fifth day on, only oils with terpene alcohols are used. In all, this treatment should last from 7 to 10 days and—if positive results are observed—should be repeated after a pause of 4 to 5 days. When using the oils containing terpene alcohols it is advantageous to alternate between different oils of this group. Those most suited for this treatment are oils with a strong antiviral, but mild, quality, such as tea

tree, peppermint, *Ravensare aromatica*, *Eucalyptus radiata*, palmarosa, niaouli, and—not really of this group but effective here—laurel.

When following these suggestions, depending on the nature of the illness, these are areas in which aromatherapy may only partially stimulate healing (see page 99). Since the treatment is harmless, however, it is certainly worth a try.

Aromatherapy and Asthma

Aromatherapy unfortunately does not offer miracle cures for today's increasing number of "civilization illnesses"—miracle cures that would remove all symptoms overnight and save us from dealing with the real causes of the problem. Nonetheless, in many cases aromatherapy does relieve symptoms. The approach of aromatherapy is multifaceted and will orient itself to the individual. For this reason, no recipes are provided. Instead, the typical methods of aromatherapy will be illustrated using the example of asthma; then these methods can be transferred to other problem areas using oils applicable for each case.[3]

The conventional medical approach for

TREATMENT PLAN FOR WEAKENED IMMUNITY

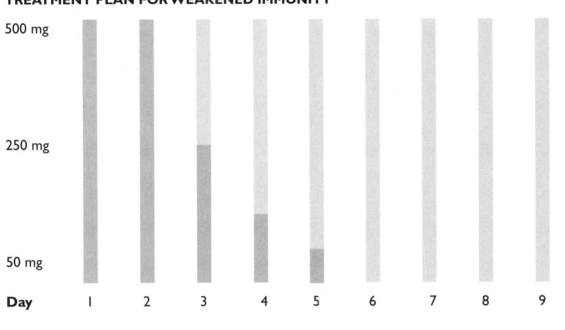

Oils containing phenol: oregano or thyme (thymol type)
Oils containing terpene alcohol (to be applied alternately): ravensare, palmarosa, *Eucalyptus radiata,* tea tree, coriander, thyme (thymol type)

Therapy for weakened immunity (according to Franchomme): After two days of intensive therapy the amount of oils containing phenol is steadily decreased while the amount of oils containing terpene alcohol is increased accordingly.

treating asthma is predominantly symptom-oriented and fairly useless with respect to the real causes of the illness. The exclusive treatment of symptoms often leads to a multilayered dependency for the patient. More often than not, patients find themselves trapped in a vicious cycle of symptom relief and negative side effects. Cortisone and other steroids, for example, often create a physical dependence.

The psychologically dependent asthma patient believes that survival is impossible without the medication. This situation is easily observed when an asthma patient suffers shortness of breath, or fears an encroaching asthma attack, and has no inhaler within reach. The stress created by not having the medication immediately at hand tends to worsen the situation.

Asthma patients often agree that they have adopted their illness into their lives as a means of communicating emotional states or desires. An integral part of any asthma treatment should therefore be to find out what a patient really wants to communicate. Often the signals sent by asthma patients express a need for attention or love. They can be of a totally different nature, however, and signify the need for more breathing room, personal space, or more distance. Perhaps the most important step to healing, or self-healing, is for the asthma patient to learn to send these signals verbally.

Sucessful reconditioning requires encouragement and support from friends and family. The psyche's influence on illnesses such as asthma and dermatitis is well known, and has been discussed more thoroughly elsewhere. Therefore, only those measures through which aromatherapy supports the healing process shall be discussed here.

Treating asthma with aromatherapy is a double-edged sword. For one, there is the danger that improper or premature treatment will have the opposite result of the intended effects. Thoughtless use of essential oils can trigger strong reactions in some patients, even a serious attack. On the other hand, there is the possibility that proper treatment with essential oils significantly aids the healing process.

Successful treatment of asthma with aromatherapy first requires distinguishing between two types of patients, depending on how far their condition has already progressed. One type of patient has long suffered from asthma and has received allopathic treatment, the other patient has experienced problems with breathing but is not yet dependent on allopathic medications.

In the first case, the illness has often already taken on a life of its own and developed into a complex pattern of physical problems requiring several phases of treatment for improvement. In the second, less serious case, the following two aromatherapy measures will most likely be suffi-

cient. In the latter case, it should be possible to limit the symptoms through a supporting and generally strengthening treatment.

Treating asthma with aromatherapy starts with familiarizing the patient with essential oils and the concept of aromatherapy. This should be a gradual and cautious process, especially if the patient has never encountered essential oils before.

A reconditioning of the way fragrances are judged is often helpful in acquainting patients with the natural qualities of essential oil fragrances. Often, people who suffer from "civilization illnesses" are exclusively used to synthetic aromas and find the purity and potency of genuine essential oils not particularly attractive. Best suited to initiate the needed reconditioning are gentle massages with essential oils whose fragrances are widely accepted and that have good spasmolytic properties. Especially recommended are lavender and mandarin oils. Tangerine oil should not be used at this stage, as it lacks the spasmolytic agent methyl anthranilate, which is found in mandarin. Other oils that harmonize with a basic blend of mandarin or lavender are Roman chamomile, spikenard, or clary sage. Experience has shown that asthma patients who react positively to these oils will soon begin to develop a positive attitude toward aromatherapy.

This first phase serves to familiarize the patient with the natural scents of essential oils as well as provide a cautious introduction to the spasmolytic qualities. The second phase focuses on the introduction of stronger oils more specifically geared to the asthma condition. Suitable choices are oils such as *Eucalyptus radiata* or *Ravensare aromatica,* which have not only expectorant qualities but—because of the presence of terpineol—surprising anti-asthmatic effects. For best results, these oils are applied freely to wet skin during or after a shower.

If a patient reacts positively to these stronger measures, a third phase geared toward easing the patient's specific symptoms can be initiated.

For patients whose asthma is attributable to the complex "nervous and allergic," spasmolytic, stabilizing mixtures of tarragon, mandarin, and rosemary (verbenone type) are recommended. This mixture can be either inhaled using a diffusor or taken orally in gelatin capsules. Other oils that can be advantageously used in this phase, depending on the patient's personality, are cypress, ylang ylang, and Roman chamomile. For patients whose asthma has turned into a more or less chronic combination of asthma and bronchitis, it is often advantageous to use stimulating oils, such as oregano, to strengthen the organism. If these measures prove successful, and the patient begins to realize that aromatherapy improves his or her condition, essential oils may then be used to treat acute attacks. Suitable for this is a mixture of two specific oils: 1 milliliter Khella (*Ammi visnaga*), and 2 milliliters creeping hyssop[4] (*Hyssopus officinalis* var. *decumbens*). Ten suppositories are made with 3 milliliters essential oil mixture in 30 grams of suppository base (cocoa butter, for example) (see page 100).

Aromatherapy and Viral Diseases

Viral diseases represent the greatest future challenge—at least in Western industrialized countries—to holistic healing methods. The multilayered mechanisms of aromatherapy have already shown that essential oils have a leading role to play. In summary:

1. The effectiveness of terpenes for emotional and physical health has been clinically proven for a long time. Very good therapeutic results have been achieved with symptoms of nervousness, anxiety, depression, inner tension, headache, dizziness, heart pains, general exhaustion, fatigue, insomnia, and loss of appetite (see chapter 3).

2. Improvement of emotional stability and mood has a pronounced influence on the ability of the immune system to defend against disease.

3. Summarizing, it can be stated that essential oils strengthen the immune response and are immediately effective against viruses (see chapter 3), a combination which explains the dynamic effectiveness of essential oils against viral illnesses.

An End to the Separation of Body and Mind

In the future, aromatherapy and other alternative methods which rely on natural substances to unite psychological and physical healing will become increasingly more important. Exciting new research in the field of psychoneuroimmunology[5] reveals a close relationship between emotional and nervous processes and the human immune system. This proves scientifically what many people have long known: the psychological constitution of a patient is of the utmost importance in the healing process. In so-called primitive societies, shamans treat the sick using pharmacological as well as psychological means. Administration of mostly plant-derived medicines is effectively coupled with a ritual reaffirming hope and belief.

Many holistic healing methods are still unjustifiably lumped into the category of quackery and hocus-pocus, but more and more science is turning to the interdependence of body and mind and is gaining insight into the control mechanisms of the brain and their influence on the emotions and the immune system. Our mind seems to be part of a remarkable communication network operating not just in the brain, but over the entire body.[6]

Considering all of this, the mechanism in which essential oils work is even more complex than has been known thus far and much more effective than that of a one-dimensional, isolated substance.

Dear Kurt,

We met each other ten years ago at an aromatherapy seminar in Paris. You had just finished studying medical aromatherapy in France to take this unique knowledge to the United States and to disseminate it in the form of your courses and by founding the Pacific Institute of Aromatherapy. You knew of me through my clinical research in the field of aromatherapy and through the 1981 compendium, *Phytomedicine*. From the first moment we were on the same wavelength and already then you invited me to come to the U.S. But at the time my family and I had just gotten visas to emigrate to Australia, and we had begun preparing for our departure in 1985. So much has happened in the past ten years, in both the world and our private lives.

Last year, at the Aroma '93 Conference in Great Britain, I was impressed with your talk on the role of essential oils for viral disease, your timely contemporary style, and your emphasis on taking back the responsibility for one's own health. It was clear to me that my own lectures on the Aromatic Revolution and the Immune System of Mankind draw their inspiration from the same source, the holistic way of thinking.

We had occasion to meet often before the conference in Brighton, and I will always be grateful for your events in the states, and for your great contribution in spreading my work there. But even before you invited me to the U.S. you had begun, indirectly, to spread the word about aromatherapy in Australia and the South Pacific. I arrived in Australia in 1986 with my family, and it didn't take long before I began meeting students of yours who had come from California to Australia having brought the knowledge you had given them. Connections between continents and cultures are getting stronger and stronger, and when the time comes to write the history of aromatherapy, your role in building new bridges will have a prominent place. When we decided to return to Europe in 1987, we knew that your students would continue our work. And indeed, in Australia today, medical aromatherapy is a strictly regulated and established therapy.

On October 27, 1988, I came to the United States for the first time. We gave a very successful seminar at the Pacific Institute of Aromatherapy in San Rafael, where we met influential personalities in the American aromatherapy movement.

In April 1989, as part of the aromatherapy symposium you sponsored, you provided one of two conference days for my presentation. On April 30, in Santa Rosa, for the first time in public I presented the basic principles of the aromatic tryptich. The ovation at the end of my presentation was proof that my concept had been understood and accepted.

Looking back at the past ten years has confirmed that your scientific training and my medical practice have much common ground, and that we each have as our mission bringing the concept of natural and effective means of maintaining our health to a wider public consisting of both specialists and laypeople.

I see the future of aromatherapy in intensified scientific research on essential oils and their medical uses, as well as in developing increased understanding of why these aromatic plant substances are so well suited for helping humans. I'm convinced that the day is not too far away when our efforts will produce results far beyond anything we would dare to imagine today. This book is most important in speeding up the necessary development of the processes of aromatherapy, in which the French–German–English triad anticipates the cooperation of the coming years.

The French approach emphasizes the medicinal and internal uses of essential oils. In England the emphasis is on external application of oils, while the German situation is somewhat paradoxical: for one, Germany is the home of active research into the medical effects of oils; on the other hand, the actual use of essential oils has not reached a corresponding level. In the U.S. the position of the Pacific Institute of Aromatherapy is probably unique. Through your seminars and medically trained guest lecturers, many American aromatherapy enthusiasts, naturopaths, and physicians became familiar with aromatherapy.

The exchange among the various forms of aromatherapy will determine its quality tomorrow. Starting in 1995, for example, I have been contracted to teach the internal applications of essential oils in England. Your book opens the way for this new quality of aromatherapy. For the energy you have invested in it, and for the seriousness of your commitment to aromatherapy, I thank you with all my heart.

Dr. Daniel Pénoël
Aouste-sur-Sye, 8 September 1994

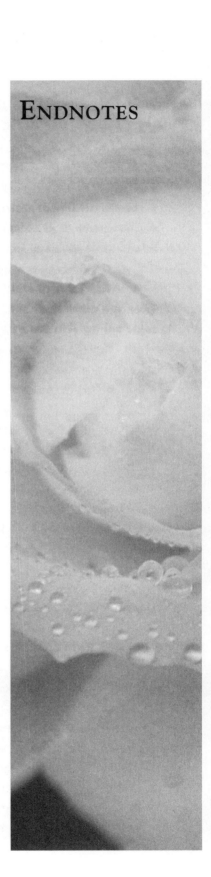

ENDNOTES

Chapter 1

1. Michael A. Schmidt, Lendon H. Smith, Keith W. Sehnert. *Beyond Antibiotics*, Berkeley, California 1993.
2. H. C. Neu. "The Crisis in Antibiotics Resistance," *Science* 257/1992, pp. 1064–73.
3. Kurt Langbein, Hans-Peter Martin, Hans Weiss, Roland Werner. *Gesunde Geschäfte*, Cologne 1982.
4. D. S. Bauman, H. E. Hagglund. "Polysystem Chronic Complainers," *Journal of Advanced Medicine*, 4(1)/1991.
5. J. D. Davidson, W. Rees-Mogg: *The Great Reckoning*, New York 1994
6. Monte Paulsen. "The Cancer Business," *Mother Jones*, San Francisco, May/June 1994, p. 41.
   Chemical firms such as the British Zeneca Group PLC make profits from such dubious drugs as Tamoxifen, a treatment for breast cancer ($470 million profit), as well as cancer-causing herbicides (Acetochlor, $300 million profit). In addition, there are also complex connections with cancer research organizations, such as the American Cancer Society, concealing the connection between these

pesticides and breast cancer, with the aid of targeted "good will" initiatives. Zeneca is the founder and sole sponsor of Breast Cancer Awareness Month in the U.S. which tried deliberately to direct public attention away from chloro-pesticides. This has certainly not had the effect that a ban on chloro-pesticides would have had. In Israel, where a ban on these pesticides has been in effect for many years, the breast cancer rates consequently fell by 8 percent.

7. Theodore Roszak. *Ökopsychologie. Der entwurzelte Mensch und der Ruf der Erde* (Original English title: Voice of the Earth), Stuttgart 1994.
8. Candace Pert. *Die chemische Kommunikation* [Chemical Communication], in Bill Moyers, Die Kunst des Heilens [The Art of Healing], Munich 1994.
9. James Gleick. *Chaos*, London 1988.
10. René-Maurice Gattefossé. *Gattefossé's Aromatherapie*, Aarau 1994.
11. Jean Valnet: *Aromatherapie*, Munich 1986.
12. Paul Belaiche. *Traité de Phytothérapie et d'Aromathérapie*, Paris 1979.

Chapter 2

1. P. M. Müller, D. Lamparsky (eds.). *Perfumes*, London, 1991.
2. All countries that establish standards have an agreement with the International Organization of Standards (ISO), which establishes binding standards for various goods (compare with the German DIN, or European EN).

3. Ernest Günther. *The Essential Oils*, New York 1948.
4. E. Gildemeister, F. Hoffmann. *Die Ätherischeh Öle*, Berlin 1956.
5. E. F. K. Denny. *Flied Distillation for Herbaceous Oils*, Tasmania, Australia 1987
6. H. Römmelt, A. Zuber, K. Dimagi, H. Drexel. *Zur Resorption von Terpenen aus Badezusätzen*, Münchner Medezinische Wochenschriften 11/1974, pp. 537–40.

   The amazing ability of essential oils to penetrate tissue has been proven repeatedly in scientific experiments. Essential oils penetrate tissue roughly 100 times faster than water and 10,000 times faster than salts.
7. P. Tétényi. "Polychemismus bei ätherischölhaltigen Pflanzenarten," *Planta Medica* 28/1975, pp. 244–56.

   R. Henauer. "Die biologische und systematische Bedeutung von chemischen Rassen," *Planta Medica* 28/1975, pp. 230–43.
8. Thymol and carvacrol are naturally occuring phenols with especially stimulating and antiseptic properties. See p. 24.
9. K. H. Kubeczka. "Möglichkeiten der Qualitätsbeurteilung arzneilich verwendeter ätherischer Öle," in *Vorkommen und Analytik ätherischer Öle*, Stuttgart 1979.
10. Actually, isoprene does not appear in nature as a free molecule, but is bound to two molecules of phosphoric acid, and is correctly known as isopentenylpyrophosphate.
11. A note on the terminology of terpenes: Terpene molecules are distinguished by

their size, that is the number of isoprene units (monoterpene, sesquiterpene, diterpene, etc.) and whether that molecule contains a functional group or not. So there are monoterpene hydrocarbons (C_{10}-molecules) and sesquiterpene hydrocarbons (C_{15}-molecules) without functional groups, as well as monoterpene and sesquiterpene alcohols, etc. In the literature a distinction between terpenes, terpene hydrocarbons and, for example, terpene alcohols is not always made. In general, the simpler "terpene" shall be used and the more precise terms such as *terpene hydrocarbons* (or *terpene alcohols*) only when necessary.

Molecule size: *terpene* and *monoterpene* are used interchangably. When referring to a structure with 15 hydrocarbon atoms, the prefix "sesqui-" is used.

12. Pierre Franchomme, Daniel Pénoël. *L'Aromathérapie exactement*, Limoges 1990.

13. H. Wagner, L. Sprinkmeyer. "Über die pharmakologische Wirkung von Mellissengeist," *Deutsche Apotheker Zeitung* 113 (30)/1973, pp. 1159–66.

14. Pierre Franchomme, Daniel Pénoël. *L'Aromathérapie exactement*, Limoges 1990.

15. V. Jakoviev, O. Isaac, K. Thiemer, R. Kunde. "Pharmakologische Untersuchungen von Kamillen-Inhaltsstoffen," *Planta Medica* 35/179, pp. 118–40.

16. There are actually four chemotypes of German chamomile: (–)α-bisabolol type (used here), α-bisabolol oxide A type, α-bisabolol oxide B type, and α-bisabolone type. The α-bisabolol oxide A is by far the most common type found in the market.

Chapter 3

1. W. Keller, W. Kober. "Möglichkeiten der Verwendung ätherischer Öle zur Raumdesinfektion," *Arzneimittelforschung* 5 (4) 1954, pp. 224–29.

2. A. M. Jansen, J. J. C. Scheffer, A. Baerheim-Svendsen. "Antimicrobial Activity of Essential Oils: A 1976–1986 Literature Review, Aspects of Test Methods," *Planta Medica* 53 (5)/ 1987, pp. 395–98

3. H. Wagner, L. Sprinkmeyer. "Über die pharmakologische Wirkung von Mellissengeist," *Deutsche Apotheker Zeitung* 113 (30)/ 1973, pp. 1159–66.

4. Paul Belaiche: *Traité de Phytothérapie et d'Aromathérapie*, Paris 1979.

5. Daniel Pénoël. "The Immune System of Mankind," *Aroma '93*, Conference Proceedings, Hove 1994.

6. G. May, G. Wilhelm. "Antivirale Wirkung wäßriger Pflanzenextrakte in Gewebekulturen," *Arzneimittel-Forschung* 28/1978, pp. 1–7.

7. A. Lembke, R. Deininger. "Wirking von Terpenen auf mikroskopische Pilze, Bakterien und Viren," in *Phytotherapie, Grundlagen—Klinik—Praxis*, Stuttgart 1987.

8. Ed Alstat. "Lomatium Dissectum, An Herbal Virucide," *Complementary Medicine* May/June 1987, pp. 32–33.

9. E. Teuscher, M. Melzig, E. Villmann, K. U. Möritz. "Untersuchungen zum Wirkungsmechanismus ätherischer Öle," *Zeitschrift für Phytotherapie* 11 (3)/ 1990, pp. 87–92.

10. E. M. Boyd, E. P. Sheppard. "The Effect of Steam Inhalation of Volatile Oils on the Output and Composition of Respiratory Tract Fluid" (nach Buchbauer und Hafner), citation in: *Pharmazie in unserer Zeit* 14 (1)/ 1985, pp. 8–18.

11. D. Schäfer, W. Schäfer. "Pharmakologische Untersuchungen zur bronchiolytischen und sekretolytisch-expektorierenden Wirksamkeit einer Salbe," *Arzneimittelforschung* 31 (1)/1981, pp. 82–86.

     H. Römmelt, W, Schnitzer, M. Swoboda, E. Senn. "Pharmakokinetik ätherischer Öe nach Inhalation mit einer terpenhaltigen Salbe," *Zeitschrift fur Phytotherapie* 9 (1)/1988, pp. 14–16.

12. K. H. Büchner, H. Hellinge, M. Huber, E. Peukert, L. Späth, R. Deininger. "Doppelblindstudie zum Nachweis der therapeutischen Wirkung von Melissengeist bei psychovegetativen Syndromen," *Medezinische Klinik* 69/1974, pp. 1032–36.

13. K. H. Lingen. "Über die therapeutische Wirksamkeit von Melissengeist bei psychovegetativen Syndromen," *Die Heilkunst* 87 (2)/1974, pp. 1–3.

14. O. Hammer. "Wirkungsnachweis zur therapeutischen Anwendung von Terpenen," *Folia phytotherapeutica* 6 (4)/ 1974.

15. H. Wagner, L. Sprinkmeyer. "Über die pharmakologische Wirkung von Melissengeist," *Deutsche Apotheker Zeitung* 113 (30)/1973, pp. 1159–66.

16. Pierre Franchomme, Daniel Pénoël. *L'Aromathérapie exactement*, Limoges 1990.

Chapter 4

1. Michael Castleman. "Legalize It," *Mother Jones*, San Francisco, December 1994, p. 46.

2. The physiological barrier between the blood vessels and the nerve cells in the brain which can only be penetrated by specific molecules.

3. Anneliese Ott. *Haut und Pflanzen*, Stuttgart 1991.

4. Jean Claude Lapraz. "Possible Side Effects of Essential Oils," *Phyto-Aromatherapy Seminar*, Los Angeles, 20 February 1993.

Chapter 5

1. It should be mentioned that experiments of this type, with regards to the procedure and the received data, have not been undisputed in the academic world. Nonetheless, they are included here as they provide a convincing correlation between the chemical nature of molecules (i.e., their tendencies to take up or donate electrons) and their basic pharmocological activity; and they establish a sensible, if somewhat rough, system of oils and their qualities which has proven itself empirically over the past ten years.

2. Perhaps the most comprehensive source of information on the current state of knowledge on the composition of essential oils is *Essential Oils 1976–1991* by Brian M. Lawrence (Carol Stream, Illinois 1993).

This is a four-volume compilation of Lawrence's regular column ("Progress in Essential Oils Research") in the journal *Perfumer and Flavorist*.

3. Pierre Franchomme, Daniel Pénoël. *L'Aromathérapie exactement*, Limoges 1990.

4. A form of white blood cells, so-called macrophages, has the ability to eliminate foreign matter such as bacteria in the bloodstream by practically consuming them. This process is called phagocytosis.

Chapter 7

1. Pierre Franchomme, Daniel Pénoël. *L'Aromatherapie exactement*, Limoges 1990.

2. J. C. Leunis. *D l'utilisation médicale des simples*, Analyse phytosociologique, Liège 1989.

3. Monika Haas, Kurt Schnaubelt. "Breathing Space," *International Journal of Aromatherapy* 4, 4/1992, pp. 13–15.

4. It is important to use only creeping hyssop (*Hyssopus officinalis* var. *decumbens*) in this case. It contains translinalol oxide, which has anti-asthmatic and tonic effects and, unlike normal hyssop, contains no toxic ketones.

5. Candace Pert. *Die chemische Kommunikation* [Chemical Communication], in Bill Moyers, Die Kunst des Heilens [The Art of Healing], Munich 1994.

6. William Poole. *Heilen durch Hoffnung*, Köln 1994.

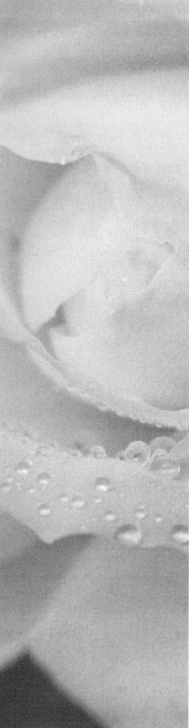

Pacific Institute of Aromatherapy

Pacific Institute of Aromatherapy
P.O. Box 6723
San Rafael, CA 94903
(415) 479-9121
Fax: (415) 479-0119

The Pacific Institute of Aromatherapy (PIA), founded in 1985 by *Advanced Aromatherapy* author Kurt Schnaubelt, Ph.D., offers educational opportunities through courses, seminars, conferences, and books. PIA offers two levels of advanced aromatherapy education: The Aromatherapy Course is a level 1 three-day certification seminar with Dr. Schnaubelt (or equivalent home study), and level 2 is the PIA Masters Program, available as home study or on location over six weekends in San Rafael.

PIA also sponsors an annual Aromatherapy Conference, bringing to light the latest in aromatherapy discoveries and knowledge; offers essential oils, including the "Travel Kit," for retail and wholesale purchase; and sells The PIA Source Book, which includes lists of producers, their oils and prices, and descriptions of the composition of essential oils in plain English.

Please contact The Pacific Institute of Aromatherapy for brochures, prices, and further information.

Suppliers

Aroma Véra (Manufacturer)
5901 Rodeo Rd.
Los Angeles, CA 90016-4312
(800) 699-9154, (310) 280-0407
Fax: (310) 280-0395
Aroma Véra offers a comprehensive line of essential oils and essential oil combinations, mostly of wild or organic origins. Its products cover skin, body, and hair care, environmental fragrancing, and gift sets and accessories, including jewelry. The company's products may be purchased at health food stores, boutiques, and salons throughout the United States and Canada, or directly from the company via mail order. The company also offers education.

Frontier Cooperative Herbs (Manufacturer)
3021 78th St.
Norway, IA 52318
(319) 227-7996, (800) 669-3275
Frontier Cooperative Herbs is one of the largest herb distributors in the United States and also offers a large selection of essential oils. Recently, Frontier Cooperative Herbs acquired Aura Cacia, another prominent aromatherapy supplier. The company's products are sold primarily through health food stores.

Original Swiss Aromatics (Manufacturer)
P.O. Box 606
San Rafael, CA 94915
(415) 479-9120
Original Swiss Aromatics offers a wide choice of essential oils, mostly of wild or organic origins, skin and body care products, and education. The company's products are available through naturopathic doctors and via mail order.

Rae Dunphy Aromatics Limited
1910 Bowness Rd. NW
Calgary, Alberta TZN 3K6
Canada
(403) 283-8889, (800) 563-8938
Rae Dunphy Aromatics, specializing in organic essential oils, carries a comprehensive range of essential oils and body care, skin care, and fragrancing products, including True Essence products, available by mail order.

RJS Inc.
Isha (Wholesale)
32422 Alipaz
San Juan Capistrano, CA 92675
(714) 240-1104, (800) 933-1008
RJS carries a comprehensive range of essential oils, available in bulk, retail and wholesale, along with diffusors and other aromatherapy accessories.

Tisserand Aromatherapy (Importer from United Kingdom)
P.O. Box 750428
Petaluma, CA 94975-0428
(707) 769-5120 (800) 227-5120
The company is named after Robert Tisserand, the author of several popular aromatherapy books and a consultant for Tisserand Aromatherapy. The company offers essential oils and skin and body care products, which can be purchased in health food stores and boutiques.

INDEX

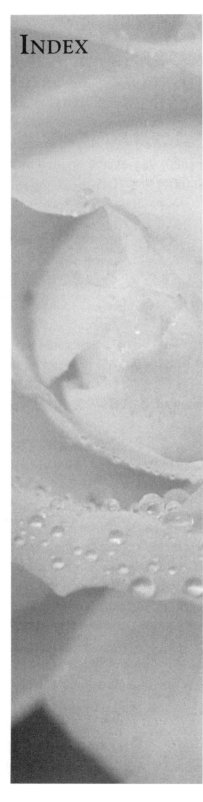